The Ethics of Health Care:
A Guide for Clinical Practice

The Ethics of Health Care:
A Guide for Clinical Practice

Raymond S. Edge, EdD, RRT
Associate Dean, College of Allied Health Sciences
Ferris State University
Big Rapids, Michigan

John Randall Groves, PhD
Assistant Professor of Humanities
Ferris State University
Big Rapids, Michigan

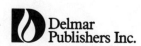
Delmar
Publishers Inc.

NOTICE TO THE READER

Cover: Timothy J. Conners

Publishing Team: David C. Gordon, Publisher
Adrianne C. Williams, Acquisitions Editor
Russell Schneck, Manager, Art, Design, & Manufacturing
Jennifer Gaines, Production Coordinator

For information, address Delmar Publishers Inc.
3 Columbia Circle
Box 15015
Albany, NY 12212-5015

Copyright © 1994 by Delmar Publishers Inc.
The ITP trademark is used under license.

Printed in the United States of America
Published simultaneously in Canada
by Nelson Canada.
a division of the Thomson Corporation

10 9 8 7 6 5 4 3 2   xxx 00 99 98 97 96 95 94

Library of Congress Cataloging-in-Publication Data

Edge, Raymond S.
   The ethics of health care : a guide for clinical practice /
Raymond S. Edge ; contributing author, John Randall Groves.
      p. cm.
   Includes bibliographical references and index.
   ISBN 0-8273-5454-1
   1. Medical ethics.   I. Groves, John Randall. II. Title.
R724.E27 1994
174'.2--dc20   93-46393
                                                                          CIP

DEDICATION

This book is dedicated to the practitioners who struggle with these issues on a daily basis. We hope that the students who read this book will join you better prepared to help you shape the future of health care.

Contents

Preface

This text is written with the allied health practitioner and nurse in mind. These specialists provide over 80 percent of the health care delivery in the United States and are often faced with dilemmas for which they have no previous educational background or experience. Not only must they deal with the ethical problems in regard to their own actions, but also they must function as members of a health care team, offering opinions, advice, and leadership.

Questions involving ethical positions are often intensely felt by those involved. These are not just armchair discussions but reach to the very heart of our perceptions of ourselves as individuals. Practitioners quickly become aware that the value given to their opinions is directly linked to the quality of the reasoning and rationales that they can provide for them. Specialists who know that something being done is wrong but cannot articulate their reasons, or the method by which they derived their beliefs, are at a real disadvantage. Not only do they fail to provide appropriate advocacy for their ideas or the patients they serve, but they also inflict upon themselves and their colleagues an incredible level of stress and discomfort.

This text is designed as a guide that takes the practitioner through a wide variety of areas involving ethical controversies. Chapters 1 through 4 present introductory materials providing a background to the study of value development and ethical theories. The reader is expected to gain an understanding of the basic principles involved in health care ethics as well as become familiar with the language by which these issues are discussed. The chapters review the major ethical systems by which these questions are being examined.

Chapter 5 provides an examination of the principle of confidentiality. Current team medicine practices create a situation where, on the average, over 75 different practitioners have legitimate access to the health care record. Many of these providers have cost-containment and reporting functions—rather than patient care—as their major concerns. In this environment, confidentiality becomes a very difficult principle to uphold.

Chapter 6 examines the subject of AIDS and the ethical problems associated with this disease. The chapter will focus on such basic issues as whether a provider has a *duty to treat* these patients. The controversy surrounding the issue of mandatory screening for patients and health care providers will be examined, as well as whether an infected health care worker can continue to practice. The need for confidentiality and respect for privacy will be discussed, as well as the conditions under which these principles are overridden by a duty to warn.

Chapter 7 examines the issues involved in withholding and withdrawing life support, and Chapter 8 presents the current controversy surrounding the modern euthanasia movement. The legal justifications for passive euthanasia and potential solutions available through the hospice movement are discussed. These chapters will be of most use to those involved in intensive and emergency care.

Chapter 9 will attempt to examine both sides of the controversial abortion issue. The authors see this issue not primarily as a health care ethics matter but rather as a social issue that has as its arena the health care setting.

Chapter 10 looks at the issues involved with the advances in genetics. This is a powerful arena for change and a new frontier for health care workers. Potential advances and uses of this new technology once again prove that Pogo was right, "The future ain't what it used to be."

Chapter 11 will examine the principle of justice as it relates to the fair and equitable distribution of health care in our society. Spiraling costs, ineffective efforts toward cost-containment, and increasing levels of maldistribution of health care benefits have all combined to make the principle of justice perhaps the most critical issue in health delivery today. The chapter will discuss how micro and macro allocation of scarce resources is undertaken according to a variety of distribution models.

Chapter 12 examines the issues of role fidelity and the requirements of professional practice. How does the nature of our specialities affect the requirements of professional practice? Issues such as disparagement of colleagues, sexual involvement with patients, scope of practice, and self-referral will be examined in light of current ethical practice.

Throughout the text, the authors provide examples of the questions that practitioners are currently facing. Where necessary, the reader will be provided a background of the legal aspects of the issues. Ours is a litigious society, and although good law may at times promote reprehensible practice, it is important to understand the current legal positions that have an impact upon health care decisions. Americans have a great respect for the law, and when there is disagreement we often seek legal clarification, even for issues involving individual values.

Clarification exercises are provided at the end of each chapter to enable the reader to explore the theoretical positions found in the material and to practice decision making. The materials are designed to enable the reader, first, to identify whether one is confronting an ethical problem. In addition, the exercises help one develop the language necessary to articulate concerns. A glossary of terms and concepts is provided for each chapter. As you come to **bold-faced words** in the material, refer to the glossary to gain a better understanding of how these words are being used.

In their works *In Search for Excellence* and *A Passion for Excellence,* Peters and Waterman state that the first step to excellence is caring. While prevention and curing provide the major focus for much of our technical training, it is the caring aspects of health provision that is the major concern of this text. As current practitioners, we have a great need for the development and furthering of the value of caring for our patients, our practice, and ourselves. However, just being concerned is not enough; concerns must be translated into appropriate language and actions. Much of the book is dedicated to teaching the language of biomedical ethics and the critical-thinking skills needed to deal with the issues. The clarification exercises will explore a variety of decision-making models. The reader will be guided though exercises that assist in gathering the facts and documenting what is occurring, identifying the ethical issues and dilemmas involved, exploring the options of initial credibility, and, finally, making and being prepared to defend the decisions.

Ethical decision making is at the very least a complex task. Practitioners must deal with facts, concepts, basic principles, and people. They must make decisions in an arena of passion, prejudice, and ambiguity. Regardless of the complexities, however, the fact remains that if we as health care providers are to be listened to as members of the health care team, it will be because we can support our views. Emotions alone—even if intensely felt and forcefully expressed in regard to an ethical problem—will not persuade others of the cogency of our views. The value attributed to our advice and decisions will be based directly on the reasoning that we have invested in the deliberative process.

Acknowledgments

The authors wish to thank all those who have assisted with the text in the areas of reading, critiquing, and arguing for change. Perhaps the greatest assistance in this area has been the work of Isabel Barnes. We have refined and shaped the clarification exercises within our classes over the last several years and therefore owe a great debt to our students for their tolerance. A debt of gratitude is owed to Jeff Ek, for his cartoons in the chapters on basic principles of abortion that helped explain the analogies used. The scenarios found in the Instructor's Manual are from Marsha Hughes and provide excellent materials for class participation. We owe a special debt to Robert Francoeur, for several of the more interesting exercises within the text— especially Grandpa's Grandpa—and for his gentle and generous encouragement over the years. The RESOLVEDD strategy is taken from the work of Raymond Pfeiffer, this decision-making matrix is both educationally useful and practical. We appreciate being able to use it in the text. As with all materials of this nature, many of our ideas for cases and problems have been borrowed and adapted from sources hidden within the mists of long discussions into a thousand evenings. To these sources we must add our thanks in the nature of the immortal words of Blanche Du Bois "Whoever you are—I have always depended upon the kindness of strangers."*

* Tennessee Williams, *A Streetcar Named Desire* (New York: New American Library, 1947).

Editorial Review Board

— CHAPTER 1 —

Human Value Development

Instructional Goal

At the end of this chapter the student should understand the nature of the human value system and relate this to the developmental theories of Lawrence Kohlberg, Jean Piaget, Morris Massey, and Carol Gilligan.

Instructional Objectives

At the end of the chapter the reader should understand and be able to:

1. Differentiate between needs and values.
2. Describe and compare the value-development positions of Massey, Kohlberg, Gilligan, and Piaget.
3. Outline the nature of the controversy found in the works of L. Kohlberg and C. Gilligan in regard to value development.
4. Describe the three general levels and six stages of value development as outlined by L. Kohlberg.
5. List the highest value levels as described by Kohlberg and Gilligan and relate them to gender development.
6. Describe the four value cohorts, as outlined by Morris Massey.
7. Explain why relativism is an inadequate basis for ethical decision making.

Glossary

1. **Altruism:** Concern for the welfare of others; selflessness.
2. **Amoral:** To be without morals; neither moral or immoral.
3. **Autonomous:** Independent, self-governing, self-determining.
4. **Egoist:** One devoted to his own self-interest and advancement.

5. **Hierarchy:** A body of graded entities, with each level subordinate to the one above.

6. **Relativist:** An individual who believes that truth is not an absolute but is relative to the individual or group that holds it.

7. **Value Cohort:** A group of individuals who experience a particular set of historical events and are value-programmed or shaped by the events as a group. For example those who experienced the great depression often shared the same values toward thrift and poverty.

8. **World View:** An individual's set of subjective values that are derived from his or her religious background, cultural heritage, and personal experiences.

NEEDS AND VALUES

The moral test of government is how it treats those who are in the dawn of life—the children; those who are in the twilight of life—the aged; and those who are in the shadows of life—the sick, the needy and the handicapped.

Hubert H. Humphrey, Vice President of the United States (1965–1969)

A major preoccupation of sages, philosophers, and social scientists throughout all ages has been a desire to understand the nature of human behavior. Although it is easy to see that human behavior is nonrandom, and designed to produce some end, it is less easy to determine the cause and effect of our actions. One useful model is to look at human behavior as a reflection of our attending to perceived needs or values.

In his classic work, Abraham Maslow listed a "**hierarchy** of needs"[1] that provide motivation for actions. According to the theory, feelings of isolation stimulate

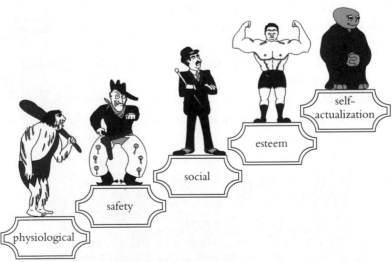

FIGURE 1–1 Hierarchy of needs

activities such as attending church or joining a bowling team, whereas hunger might stimulate food gathering. Under most situations, our actions are explainable in that we are seen as attempting to satisfy a given set of needs. According to Maslow, as each need level is satisfied, the needs of the next level become the dominant motivators for our actions. If the hierarchy of needs is correct, an observer who could determine which level of need was operational could predict the nature of our next actions (Fig. 1–1).

There are times, however, when the individuals appear to move from needs-based motivation to attending to an inner subjective set of feelings, attitudes, beliefs, and opinions that make up their personal value system. In these cases, the individuals seem to ask themselves not what they would do but rather what they should do, and the outcome is less predictable. In some sense, the difference is that found in Hume's law, which holds that there is an unbridgeable gap between fact and value, or as it is classically portrayed between "is" and "ought."[2] The facts of the physical universe can tell us what is, but it is our values that guide us to an understanding of what ought to be as it relates to human behavior. Figure 1–2 lists values that are important to our everyday choices in regard to health care. The list is by no means complete, and each individual's experiences will shape the way these values will be considered in personal decision making. Consider how a patient who placed a high value on personal independence, self-determination, personal privacy, and freedom from disability might react to a spinal injury that left him paralyzed and in need of his bodily functions being cared for by others. It is conceivable that someone might view the loss of these characteristics of the "good life" as being so important that the option of no life might be preferable. The same injury to another individual with a differing set of values—perhaps including a view that this life is a mere test for rewards given in an afterlife—might lead that person to cling to life with great tenacity, never considering death as a viable option.

To see how different a value system is from that of a needs system, one need only look at the conduct of the male passengers during the sinking of the *Titanic*. Obviously their need for survival might have motivated a host of actions such as

Independence – Freedom from constraint
Autonomy – Self-determination
Privacy/confidentiality – Fear of invasion
Self-esteem – Need to value oneself
Well-being – Freedom from pain and suffering
Security – Control of fear and anxiety
Sense of belonging – Group identification
Sexual and spiritual support – Fulfillment
Freedom from Disability – Physical/mental capacity
Accomplishment – Personal fulfillment

FIGURE 1–2 Common Decision-shaping Values

forcing their way onto the lifeboats. However, the predominate value of the time was that men should protect women and children. Therefore, as the ship went down, the bands played and the men stood aside even at the peril of their lives. Similarly, the health-care providers who sacrifice some level of personal safety to work with contagious patients and the mother who takes on the 250-pound bully in the park to protect her children are acting from a position of value, and are making decisions based on a feeling about what one ought to do.

VALUE DEVELOPMENT

Where then do we receive our values? As humans we are born with a series of undifferentiated potentials. As an example, we have the capability to learn a language, but the particular language is not proscribed by our genetic heritage. In this same sense humans have the innate capacity to acquire ethical beliefs. But the value system that we develop is dependent upon the cultural framework in which we live. This capacity to become ethical beings and to conform to some universal principles of mutual cooperation and **altruism** seems as old as the species itself. One of the earliest found skeletal remains of Neanderthal man was that of an individual, approximately 50 years of age, whose bones indicate that he suffered from a severe, debilitating form of arthritis. His impediment made it unlikely that he could hunt or engage in strenuous activity, and he, therefore, was dependent upon the caring of his group for his survival. While Neanderthal man may not have had the words to express such concepts as love, altruism, and individual respect, he seemingly exhibited behaviors by which these terms are defined.

In that we are born into this world without a prescribed set of rules for what we should do in any given situation, value development is a product of our interactions with our cultural environment. The foremost theorists in value development are Jean Piaget[3] and Lawrence Kohlberg.[4] Both Piaget and Kohlberg stress that value development is intimately tied to the individuals cognitive and psychomotor development. In their models, they describe the individual as growing through several stages of value orientation. Figure 1–3 shows the three stages of Kohlberg's model and the source of value orientation.

The Piaget model for development lists four stages, from the **amoral** infant to the **autonomous** adult, with each stage occurring at certain general ages. The Kohlberg model is very similar to that of Piaget except that it ignores the amoral phase of the infant and expands on three general levels of development (preconventional, conventional, and postconventional) and further subdivides each level into two stages. In the model, the individual matures through six phases from a value orientation based on punishment and obedience to a final autonomous stage characterized by a universal ethical orientation.

Kohlberg's Stage Theory of Moral Reasoning

Preconventional (ages 2 to 7). During this period, the child responds to the prevailing cultural values of right and wrong, good and evil. In the earliest stage of this level, the child has no real understanding of the values themselves and accepts the

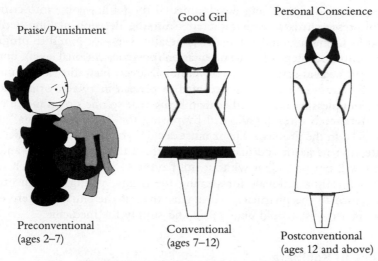

FIGURE 1–3 Orientation of Stages

authority of others. The physical consequences of the actions determine the right-ness or wrongness, regardless of the attribution of value. During the second stage, the child will begin to direct his or her activities toward the satisfaction of personal needs, rather than the needs of others. Human relations are viewed in terms of the marketplace, and are interpreted in a physical, pragmatic way, not in terms of loyalty or justice. Some **egoist** theories hold that this stage, where the individual is focused on personal satisfaction, is all there is to morality.

Conventional (ages 7 to 12). At this point, the child conforms to societal expecta-tions of family, group, or nation in order to win the approval of authority figures. Stage one includes a form of good boy/good girl orientation as the child seeks to conform to expected social conventions. Good behavior pleases or helps others; one earns approval by being nice and having good intentions. During stage two of this level, the focus becomes fixed on the rules, social order, and respect for authority. During this time, right behavior consists of doing one's duty, social order, and showing respect for authority. "My country right or wrong" would have meaning at this level of development.

Postconventional (age 12 and above). The focus of this level is the development of the social contract and autonomous decisions apart from outside authorities. In the first stage, the child establishes a social-contract orientation and attempts to conform to the ever-changing values and demands of society. In the final stage of value development, abstract qualities such as justice and respect for the rights and dignity of others become important, and one's conscience becomes the final arbiter in regard to ethical dilemmas. Essentially, the individual subscribes to a set of abstract, but universal, principles such as justice, humane reciprocity, respect for the dignity of the individual, and equality. At this point, the individual is essentially morally autonomous, and decides what is right through personal conscience.

In recent years, the Kohlberg developmental model has come into criticism, as most of his research data were gathered from the decision-making activities of young males. Using his model, females generally were not found to progress into the final autonomous stage of value orientation (postconventional level), but seemed arrested in the second stage of the conventional level. Instead of becoming essentially morally autonomous, females seemed to plateau in a value orientation based on helping and pleasing others rather than being true to one's own moral compass.

This difference is often highlighted by posing the "Heinz dilemma" to young boys and girls. In the problem, Heinz must decide whether to steal medicine for his dying wife after he has found that he cannot afford the purchase price and that the pharmacist will not provide it without full payment. While young men will often work out a legalistic rationale for stealing the drugs, young women often want Heinz to return to the pharmacist, believing that, if the situation were explained better, the pharmacist would understand and supply the medicine.

Challenges to Kohlberg

Carol Gilligan[5] has challenged the Kohlberg model and the assumption that males and females see value problems in the same light. One interesting aspect of her research was the study of boys and girls at play. Boys tended to play longer and more complicated games than girls, and, during play, often settled disputes by arguing out a set of rules under which the game could go forward. Girls, on the other hand, seemed to play games with fewer rules and ended a game when disputes developed. The rationale given for this difference was that boys were willing to subordinate relationships to rules and principles, while girls were not. Gilligan argues for a separate value-development pathway for females that results in a different highest value, personal responsibility for females, and legalistic equality for males.

It is interesting to note that the difference observed by Gilligan is somewhat confirmed by the typographical profile created by Isabel Myers and Katherine Briggs[6] which looks at normal human behavior. Men and women score equally on all the major dimensions of the instrument with the exception of decision making. In this area, men fall predominately within the "thinking" category for decision making, being more comfortable with following rules, laws, formulas, and the like, and subordinating relationships to principles. Women, on the other hand, are more likely to fall into the "feeling" category, where decisions are based on relationships and personal outcomes rather than on legalisms and rules. Whether this is truly a difference between men and women, or just a function of what has been fostered by our culture, is yet to be determined and will become more clear as the traditional roles of the sexes are further blurred. (Figure 1–4 indicates how each of these decision-making methods is perceived by others.) Thinking and feeling are just two described methods of making decisions—neither being preferred or useful in all situations. Unfortunately, as a culture we have only recently begun to value the feeling method of decision making. Everyone uses both approaches; however females predominantly use the feeling pathway and males the thinking pathway.

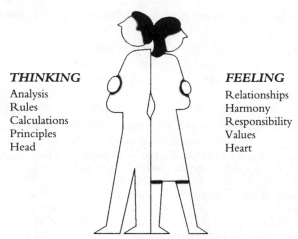

THINKING
Analysis
Rules
Calculations
Principles
Head

FEELING
Relationships
Harmony
Responsibility
Values
Heart

FIGURE 1–4 Modes of Decision Making: Men and women use both thinking and feeling as methods; however men prefer the thinking mode and women prefer feeling.

Massey's Value Cohorts

This rather subjective screen of feelings, attitudes, beliefs, and opinions with which we view and judge our world is taught to us by our early environment. According to some value theorists, the critical period of value programming is between birth and teens, with approximately 90 percent of our value system being firmly in place by age ten. Beyond this age, our general values rarely change unless we are affected by some significant emotional event. The value theorist Morris Massey[7] uses the phrase "you are what you are because of where you were when" to emphasize that we are programmed by events that occurred around us as we were growing up. In that certain events happen to us as a group, these shape us as a generational **value cohort**. An excellent example of cohort programming can be seen in the population that was young during the great depression of the 1930s. As a group, this is a very security-conscious portion of our population. Whether real or imagined, the ideas of doing without, or "walking five miles through the snow to school," or "a penny saved is a penny earned" are important to them, and yet these notions seem almost mythic to that portion of the population born after 1940.

In his work, Massey describes four general value cohorts programmed by the events of recent national history. Figure 1–5 shows the **world view** orientation of the four value cohorts. Although some individuals may escape the impact of certain eras (for example a hermit may escape the impact of urbanization, and the idle rich may escape economic downturns), most in the society will be shaped and programmed by the value-molding forces around them. The major current generation clusters identified by Massey are broken down into four broad categories of world view value differences:

   1. Traditionalists. This group received their value programming by the events of the 20s, 30s, and early 40s—a period when family structure was extended, and clearly identified roles were still in place. The war traditionalists fought was generally

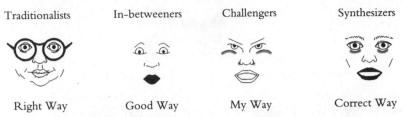

FIGURE 1–5 World View of the Value Cohorts

successful and popular. As a result, this group tends toward patriotism as well as the recognition of authority and legitimate chain of command. Several periods of economic scarcity were included in this time era, leaving the group with a certain level of materialism based on the concept that "whatever" we do without as we grow up is important to us."

According to Massey, Traditionalists have been shaped to believe in a set of prescribed codes of action that determine how a person behaves on the job, at home, and socially. For them, society is best structured with everyone knowing, and being in, his or her appropriate place. In some way, they view life as a team sport in which all the players should support the action and be happy in their assigned roles. Even wildly popular cultural heroes such as Generals Patton and MacArthur could not escape their assigned roles and suffered when they were considered non–team players.

Several cultural trends over the last decades—such as the decline of the work ethic, the loss of defined family roles, and the emergence of minority groups—have seriously undermined and challenged traditionalist values. This value cohort seems somewhat dislocated in time as we prepare to enter the next century. Traditionalists still, however, form much of what we recognize as the "establishment" and are in positions to make decisions that affect all of us.

2. In-Betweeners. The values shared by this cohort were those commonly programmed in the late 40s and 50s. This group is caught between the traditional values of the pre-40s and the highly individual values expressed after the mid-60s, when concepts of structure and set roles were in disarray. They seem caught between the values expressed in the phrases "I am a company man," and "You can take this job and shove it." The dynamics of being between these two polar views have left them uncomfortable with either end of the spectrum. This allows the In-Betweeners to recognize and accept regulations, but also to make calculating assessments in regard to their personal needs. In their work lives, they often appear more like the Traditionalist, conforming to standard dress and protocol, while in their private lives they may lead very individualistic and informal lifestyles.

In an attempt to maintain individuality within structure, In-Betweeners often shift between conformity and experimentation. This pursuit of a personal place leads this group to be the major consumers of the "How to be _____ books." One of their great values to society is their ability to speak the language of both the pre-40s and post-60s, thereby forming a bridge of understanding between two very different value-orientation cohorts.

3. Challengers. This cohort shares the basic programming of the early 60s through mid-70s. They are the products of a period of wealth and power. Just as scarcity made the Traditionalists somewhat materialistic, this group appears to take for granted and to devalue the world of abundance. Challenge to authority and societal values, informal dress and experimental lifestyles are all hallmarks of this cohort.

Challengers were programmed in a period of permissiveness, when individuality was prized above team play. As a result, they appear to challenge standards unless conformity benefits their own personal requirements. In organizations, they expect and demand participation and personal consideration. It is these demands for consideration of individual needs that have been the impetus for such personnel packages as flextime, employer day-care centers, pregnancy leave for men, and similar benefits.

4. Synthesizers. This is the latest of the value cohorts described in Massey's works—the programming period from the late 70s onward. This group has borrowed something from each of the three preceding value cohorts. They are more conservative than Challengers, yet more cynical and skeptical than either Traditionalists or In-Betweeners. The Synthesizers perceive a finite and perhaps shrinking world, where the future may well hold less for them in both a qualitative and quantitative sense.

Unlike the Challengers before them, the Synthesizers see the system as both the problem and the solution. They appear to accept the role of adapting to change and the creation of new systems that both provide and sustain.

Individually, we possess an organized system of thoughts, feelings, opinions, and beliefs (world view) with which we screen the events occurring around us. It is with this subjective screen, based on our culture and life experiences, that we judge the rightness or wrongness of actions as they pertain to what a person should do in a given situation. Whether individuals feel comfortable taking pens from work, pushing to the front of a line, buying goods beyond their needs, or listening quietly as elders speak is a reflection of their particular world view and value programming.

SUMMARY

In his book, *The Closing of the American Mind,*[8] Allan Bloom proposes that students entering the university may come from the left or right in regard to political views but will almost always share the position that truth is relative. This proposition is based on an accommodation to a pluralistic culture. History is viewed as a past in which men thought that they possess the truth, and in the name of this truth justified outrageous persecutions, wars, slavery, xenophobic racism, and even witch burning. The point that these students take from this reading of history is that the "true believer" is a dangerous person, and that only as we are able to avoid thinking that ours is the one right way can we survive. Openness and tolerance have become for these students the only plausible stance in the face of various claims to truth and an appropriate lifestyle. With this belief in relativism, the rational person then would not be concerned with correcting the mistakes from the past but rather would decide that all truth is relative and one view is equal to all other views.

In some sense, Massey subscribes to ethical relativism, a view that holds that there are no universal or absolute principles that bind human beings, and that the standards of right or wrong are always relative to the society or culture. In this light, the rightness or wrongness of customs or traditions that allow the placing of the aged on an ice floe to die, or the obligation of a brother to marry his dead brother's widow, could only be examined in reference to the Arctic Eskimo or African cultures from which they spring. The **relativist** would hold that there is no basis for saying that a particular act is right or wrong, independent of its cultural framework. Whatever we might believe in regard to relativism, and the lack of perfect truth, it would still seem reasonable that if we were in a position to do so, we would stop cannibals from eating missionaries and families from burning widows.

Few health care practitioners would be comfortable in taking a relativistic view of values. The decisions we must make are of such significance that the flip of a coin will not do. Some answers truly are better than others, and some decisions must not be made. To take an amoral position that somehow all answers to moral questions are equal would be unacceptable in health care practice. The philosopher Nietzsche was correct in his declaration that we are valuing animals. However, in regard to our values, humans are not programmed, as is the beast of the forest, to a proscribed set of correct actions but are condemned to lives of freedom and choice. In the practice of health care a position of "anything goes" is unacceptable. John Steinbeck, in his book *Of Mice and Men,* pointed out how bankrupt we had become in regard to moral values when one of his characters commented, "There's nothing wrong anymore."[9]

This book is about the process of choice making in the value-laden area of health care. The purpose is to provide the practitioner with the conceptual framework and language skills needed to examine value issues, and to look at a series of systems that are currently employed in making these difficult decisions. Modern health care is currently overflowing with value choices that must be made, and the choices we make will determine to a great extent the shape of our careers and the pleasure we derive from the services we perform. There is a tradition of practice whereby health care providers will not conduct themselves in an egoist manner, but will consider the needs of the patients and the profession. Our patients are filled with expectations that we will perform in an ethical manner, even if it is unclear to them and us exactly what that entails.

Value theorists, such as Lawrence Kohlberg, Jean Piaget, and Carol Gilligan, have investigated the development of these world views and have provided multi-staged models that show maturation and acquisition of value orientation throughout our childhood. The highest level of maturation described by Kohlberg and Piaget seems to be an autonomous decision-making system based upon legalistic equality. In recent years, Carol Gilligan has provided a feminist perspective and argues for separate developmental pathways for men and women, with the highest value for women being personal responsibility.

This text is not an answer book that will provide you with comfortable solutions to these tough issues, for in truth there are no easy answers. This is a book that seeks to provide you with the right questions, so that you are at least comfortable that the issue has been examined appropriately. The value placed on our opinions as nurses and allied health practitioners will be based not upon our intense feelings but rather upon the quality of the reasoning that has gone into the process.

CLARIFICATION EXERCISES

A. Massey holds that certain significant emotional events shape generational cohorts in such a way that they have a unified world view or shared value patterns. Consider the Traditionalists, the group that was value programmed in the 30s and 40s. The significant events were the depression, World War II, extended family structures, and the rise of America as a world power. Describe how you think these events might have created a common value structure toward the following:

1. Patriotism
2. Value of work
3. Family member roles
4. Cooperative Action

• Consider that this value cohort participated in a popular and successful war against seemingly evil groups. The end result of this has been a strong feeling toward national pride, and priority placed on the need for an adequate defense.

• Select someone you know who was involved in the World War II period and think of how he or she feels about patriotism, work, family roles, and cooperative action. Is the person like or unlike the generalizations you created?

• Imagine a time and place in which children are brought up (programmed) in a situation where these circumstances are common: single-parent families, poverty, no meaningful work, violent streets where people drive by and kill strangers, inadequate school systems where children enter through a metal detector, and popular media that panders to a nightmarish mixture of sexuality, violence and consumerism. Describe how you think the above might create a common world view set of values toward the following:

1. Patriotism
2. Family member roles
3. Value of work
4. Cooperative Action

B. In the next case, make your decision first using legalistic equality (male pathway) as the highest value, and then using responsibility and relationships (female pathway) as the highest value.

The case involves a man, his wife, his mother, and his son. The family is out in a boat and the man is needed to hold the tiller in order to keep the boat steady. A great wind comes in and the boat begins to founder. It becomes obvious that someone must leave the boat and drown to save the lives of the others. In that the man is needed to hold the tiller or all must perish, which of the others (the mother, son, or wife) should be sacrificed?

Legalistic equality must involve the following of rules or principles, while responsibility must be shown to take into consideration the impact on the lives of the individuals involved.

C. Beginning each statement with "A person should," write a value statement that corresponds to your views in regard to the following areas:

1. Family
2. Work
3. Honesty
4. Abortion
5. Confidentiality

D. Massey identified four different value groups, which he called Traditionalists, In-Betweeners, Challengers, and Synthesizers. Identify which of the value cohorts is best associated with the following value statements:

1. "People should know the rules and follow them." _____
2. "People can and should make caring choices that will result in a better world for all of us." _____
3. "It is a jungle out there, and he who hesitates is last." _____
4. "Life is to be explored and works best when we treat others as we would like to be treated." _____
5. "My country right or wrong." _____
6. "If you don't take care of number one, you deserve what you get." _____

REFERENCES AND SUGGESTED READING

1. Abraham Maslow, *Motivation and Personality,* rev. R. Frager, J. Fadiman, C. McReynolds, and R. Cox (New York: Harper and Row, 1987).
2. David Hume, *A Treatise of Human Nature,* ed. L. A. Selby-Bigge (Oxford: Oxford University Press, 1988).
3. Jean Piaget, *The Moral Judgment of a Child,* Trans. M. Gabain (New York: The Free Press, 1964).
4. Lawrence Kohlberg, *Philosophy of Moral Development* (San Francisco: Harper and Row, 1981).
5. Carol Gilligan, *In a Different Voice* (Cambridge, MA: Harvard University Press, 1982).
6. Isabel Myers, *Gifts Differing* (Palo Alto, CA: Consulting Psychological Press, 1980).
7. Morris Massey, as cited in Michael O'Connor and S. Merwin, *Mysteries of Motivation* (Carlson Learning Company, 1988).
8. Allan Bloom, *The Closing of the American Mind* (New York: Simon and Schuster, 1987).
9. John Steinbeck, *Of Mice and Men,* (New York: Modern Library, 1937).

CHAPTER 2

Decision Making in Value Issues

Instructional Goal

In this chapter the reader will examine the common theories and methods used in making value decisions.

Instructional Objectives

At the end of this chapter the reader should understand and be able to:

1. List the theorists who are considered the fathers of contemporary duty-oriented and consequence-oriented reasoning.
2. Outline the theoretical position known as utilitarianism, and analyze a clinical problem following its framework.
3. Outline the theoretical position of Kant, and analyze a clinical problem following his duty-oriented reasoning.
4. Differentiate between act and rule utilitarianism. State how rule utilitarianism is similar to duty-oriented reasoning.
5. List the major criticisms of duty-oriented and consequence-oriented systems.
6. Outline the theoretical position known as virtue ethics, and name the contemporary theorist associated with this position.
7. List the major criticisms of the virtue ethics position.
8. List several sources from which basic principles have been derived by duty-oriented theorists.

Glossary

Act Utilitarianism: The doctrine that skips any reference to principles and rules and judges the right action as the one that brings the greatest happiness to the greatest number.

Agape: Love for humanity, general goodwill.

Biographical Life: Life in the sense of events, and the ability to have relationships.

Classism: The doctrine that holds that one particular social class of persons is superior to another.

Consequence-oriented System: An ethical system holding that the right action is one that maximizes some good. The right thing to do in the end is based on what is the good thing to do. One cannot know what is right without an examination of the consequences.

Duty-oriented System: An ethical system that holds that the right action is one that is based on ethical principles that are known to be right, independent of whether they serve good ends.

Equal Consideration of Interest: The rule that the interests of all individuals must be considered equally. This rule, if adopted, reduces the harm and scapegoating possible in ethical systems such as utilitarianism.

Euthanasia: An easy death; the act of killing or permitting death without suffering.

Hedonism: The doctrine that the chief good of humans lies in the pursuit of pleasure.

Mean: The moderate position, the position between extremes.

Morality: The doctrine of moral duties; quality of an action in regard to right and wrong.

Principle of Utility: The principle that holds that the right action is the one leading to satisfaction of those desires that the individual prefers to have satisfied.

Rule Utilitarianism: The doctrine that certain rules have been found to have a high utility, that is, have brought about the greatest happiness for the greatest number. The rule utilitarian justifies actions by appealing to these universal rules such as "Do not steal," which are in turn justified by the principle of utility.

Utilitarianism: The doctrine that utility is the sole standard of moral conduct; the doctrine of the greatest happiness for the greatest number.

VALUE CONFRONTATIONS

This is the heyday of the ethicist in medicine. He delineates the rights of patients, of experimental subjects, of fetuses, of mothers, of animals, and even of doctors. (And what a far cry it is from the days when medical "ethics" consisted of condemning economic improprieties such as fee splitting and advertising!) With impeccable logic— once certain basic assumptions are granted—and with graceful prose, the ethicist develops his arguments . . . Yet his precepts are essentially the product of armchair exercise and remain abstract and idealistic until they have been tested in the laboratory of experience.

F.J. Ingelfinger, M.D.

As practitioners, we are educated in the science and art of our specialties. Questions in regard to drug preparations, pathologic entities, and appropriate therapeutics often seem to have straightforward and comfortable answers. We know that, if we apply the right set of equations or follow the correct procedures, a best answer comes forward. These answers are often reproducible and can be verified, and one need only present the facts in order for everyone to come into agreement. Yet health care is also an arena where values play a commanding role in what is right and good for our patients. Unfortunately for all practitioners, in the arena of values there is often disagreement, and rarely are the answers comfortable.

It is our values that tell us what is right and wrong, good and evil, and that imply a preference in regard to correct human behavior. This rather subjective screen with which we surround ourselves often countenances strong feelings or intense attitudes that are backed by rational justifications. Although we tend to think of value problems in the "big ethics" sense—i.e. those problems that are involved in choices dealing with life and death—we are also bedeviled by rather everyday questions that call for judgment based on a perception of right and wrong.

Is it right or wrong to take a gift from a patient? Is it acceptable to own a portion of a diagnostic clinic to which you refer patients? Should a pharmacist criticize a physician who will not change a drug order even though the order is clearly not in the best interest of the patient? What is the nurse's duty when another nurse makes an error? Should you tell a patient who asks about the quality of specific medical care that in your opinion the physician is a jerk? If you gave a treatment to the wrong patient, but did not harm the patient in the process, do you have to confess the error? As a physical therapist, if the patient could not afford the care but needed it, would it be OK to falsify insurance papers in order to provide the appropriate care for your patient? As a respiratory therapist, would it be OK to accept a finder's fee from a home health equipment company to which you referred your hospital patients? Whereas none of these questions involves life or death decisions, they call for value choices and are subject to very different answers depending upon the value structure of the practitioner.

Perhaps the most frustrating aspect of value choices is that honorable individuals often come to very different positions based on reasoning from their particular world views. Some will base their opinions on formal philosophical or religious beliefs, while others will try to weigh the potential outcomes—seeking to chose those that provide the greatest good for the greatest number. Still others really don't use a formal system at all to determine the right answer but will rely upon current practice or past experiences as their guides.

In that values are not subject to scientific analysis or deal with items that are NOT easily quantifiable, value arguments are often deeply felt and rarely won. Because of the intense feelings associated with our values, we often come to believe that those with opposing views are not only wrong but somehow evil in their wrongness. It is in the arena of values where we often see the individual taking a stand and acting as a majority of one. As professionals, it is necessary, even in our opposition, to attempt to be constructive, not destructive, in the methods we use when we come to disagreements over issues involving personal values. For example, accommodation in regard to the issue of abortion might be more easily attained if each side had not cast the other as "baby killers" or "antiwomen."

To acknowledge that individuals can come to different opinions in regard to value issues is not to say that all opinions have the same worth or credibility, or that no particular answer is better than another. Often we will find ourselves with no "right" answer or several "right" answers that seem to fit the situation. In order to make better value decisions, we must often move beyond our initial thoughts and feelings in regard to these basic issues and to build a framework for examining them. Several theoretical positions have been proposed that allow us to examine issues that are value laden.

Although world views are individual, certain traits have been described and allow generalizations across individuals and groups. In all cultures there are a variety of common world views and ethical systems. One polar dichotomy found is that of the **consequence-oriented** and **duty-oriented** world views and theories.

TELEOLOGICAL (CONSEQUENCE-ORIENTED) THEORIES

Consequence-oriented theories judge the rightness or wrongness of decisions based upon outcomes, or predicted outcomes. Those following a consequence-based theory would decide that what is right also maximizes some good. The right thing to do, then, is the good thing to do. These theorists may argue about what constitutes the good, but once agreed they would have no problem, theoretically, in deciding upon a right course of action. In their works focused on the health care setting, T.L. Beauchamp and L.B. McCullough offer health (prevention, elimination, or control of disease), relief from unnecessary pain and suffering, amelioration of disabling conditions, and the prolongation of life as intrinsic goods.[1] Figure 2–1 lists a variety of consequences that have been claimed as intrinsic goods.

Jeremy Bentham and John Stuart Mill[3] are considered the fathers of **utilitarianism,** the most common form of consequence-oriented reasoning. To a utilitarian, the good resides in the promotion of happiness, or the greatest net increase of pleasure over pain. The purest form of this line of reasoning is **act utilitarianism,** where the decision is based on listing the possible alternatives for action, weighing each in regard to the amount of pleasure or utility it provides, and selecting the course of action that maximizes pleasure. There is some criticism that this **hedonistic** form of reasoning might lead to situations in which one group derives pleasure from the pain of others and justifies their actions on the basis of utility. To overcome this objection, some newer consequentialist formulations have required that the principle of **equal consideration of interest** be shown, where the individual is not allowed to increase his share of happiness at the expense of another. Each person's happiness must be considered equally. One of the real problems of act utilitarianism is that the individual must somehow predict and calculate the various levels of happiness promoted by each choice. In the worst-case usage of utilitarianism, individuals might be seen to shift from one position to another as they weigh the

Proposed Intrinsic Goods

- life, consciousness, and activity
- health and strength
- pleasure and satisfaction of all or certain kinds
- happiness, beatude, contentment
- truth
- knowledge and true opinion of various kinds, wisdom
- beauty, harmony, proportion in objects contemplated
- aesthetic experience
- morally good dispositions or virtues
- mutual affection, love, friendship, cooperation
- just distribution of goods and evils
- harmony and proportion in one's own life
- power and experiences of achievement
- self-expression
- freedom
- peace, security
- adventure and novelty
- good reputation, honor, esteem (2)

FIGURE 2–1

various levels of happiness and pain avoidance and, in the process, lose their sense of self.

Utilitarian systems are referred to as teleological theory, taken from the Greek word *telos,* which means end. The basic concept is that the right act is that which brings about the best outcome. Often, individuals will attempt to use utilitarian theory when they seek to divide scarce resources such as health care. They might justify the denial of a single individual access to a heart transplant if the money could be spent on providing vaccine for thousands. Figure 2–2 is a flow chart model of how decisions are made using a utilitarian system.

Criticisms of Utilitarianism

1. The calculation of all the possible consequences of our actions, or worse yet our inactions, appears impossible.
2. Utilitarianism may be used to sanction unfairness and the violation of rights. In order to maximize one person's or one group's happiness, it may be necessary to infringe on the happiness of another individual or group.
3. Utilitarianism is not sensitive to the agent-relativity of duty. We are inclined to think that parents are obligated to care for their children, and that physicians are wrong to harm patients. Both of these examples could be allowed under utilitarianism, if doing so maximized overall utility.
4. Utilitarianism does not seem to give enough respect to persons. Under this theory, the ends justify the means, so it may be moral to use a person merely as a means to our ends.

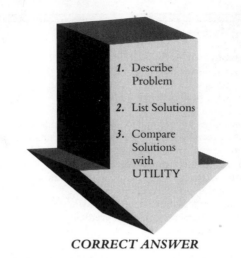

CORRECT ANSWER

FIGURE 2–2 Consequence-oriented Reasoning

5. Under utilitarianism, it is justifiable to prevent others from doing what we believe to be harmful acts to themselves. Such a paternalistic view could justify unacceptable governmental intervention into the private lives of individuals.
6. Utilitarianism alone does not provide a basis for our own moral attitudes and presuppositions. If followed, utilitarianism may recommend behaviors that are in conflict with personal fundamental moral beliefs and give rise to a sense of loss of self.

A formulation of utilitarianism that seems to avoid the problem of exact quantification required in act utilitarianism is **rule utilitarianism.** This theory holds that an action can be deemed to be right if it conforms to a rule that has been validated by the **principle of utility.** The principle of utility requires that the rule bring about positive results when generalized to a wide variety of situations. Rules forbidding the abridgment of free speech or the forceful housing of military in private homes might qualify as suitable, even if under certain rare situations they might bring about a decrease in happiness or pleasure. Consequence-oriented viewpoints are often very persuasive in that they give comfort to our modern cynicism in regard to absolute truths, also speak to our better selves in respect to tolerating the views and cultures of others. This is especially true in such recent formulations of utilitarianism as Joseph Fletcher's situation ethics[4], where the good is **agape,** which can be defined as general goodwill or love for humanity. He holds that, in the final analysis, human need determines what is or is not ethical. If an act helps people (it is a good act); if it hurts (it is a bad act).

In his writings, Fletcher provides six guidelines for making ethical choices:

1. Compassion for people as human beings
2. Consideration of consequences
3. Proportionate good
4. Priority of actual needs over ideal or potential needs
5. A desire to enlarge choice and reduce chance

6. A courageous acceptance of the need to make decisions and the equally courageous acceptance of the consequences of our decisions

As can be seen, the six guidelines provide for no appeal to an absolute principle, no authority that one can rely upon; the only possible test of rival solutions lies in the consequences. This proposal is similar to the clinical model of medicine, where the best therapeutic regime choice is the one most likely to result in an improvement in patient well-being.

DEONTOLOGICAL (DUTY-ORIENTED) THEORIES

Duty-oriented ethicists feel that the basic rightness or wrongness of an act depends upon its intrinsic nature rather than upon the situation or the consequences. This position is often described as a deontological theory, taken from the Greek word for duty. An act in itself would either be right or wrong; It could not be both. This particular world view is codified in several major ethical systems and religions. In the classic work *Groundwork of the Metaphysic of Morals,* Immanuel Kant[5] held that the consequences of an action were essentially irrelevant. Kant based his moral philosophy on the crucial fact that we are rational beings, and a central feature of this rationality was that principles derived from reason were universal. He held that morality is derived from rationality, not from experience, and that obligation is grounded not in the nature of man or in the circumstances of the world but in pure reason. These universal truths applied to all people, for all times, in all situations. Kant held that the human mind works the same way, regardless of who you are, where you are, or when you are. An action could be known to be right when it was in accordance with a rule that satisfied a principle he called a categorical imperative. By "categorical" he meant they do not admit exceptions. An "imperative" is a command derived from a principle. These imperatives were formulated by finding a maxim that could be understood as universal law. The imperatives seem to have three elements; (1) universal application, i.e. binding upon every individual, (2) unconditionally, and (3) demanding an action. An example of this might be the unconditional duty of a lifeguard to enter the water to save a drowning man. The mental process for the lifeguard would be a series of questions, "Should all paid lifeguards attempt to rescue drowning individuals?" "Is this duty to rescue unconditional?" and, finally, "Does this particular incident require the actions of a lifeguard?" If the lifeguard answered yes to all three questions, according to Kant he would have a binding moral duty to act.

One such maxim relevant to health ethics is; "We must always treat others as ends and not as means only." Kant saw people as having an absolute value based upon their ability to make rational choices. Accordingly, our dignity was derived from this capacity, and this was violated whenever a person was treated merely as a means to an end (a thing) and not as a person. From this one maxim you could derive the other principles used in the ethics of health care. An action, then, could be judged right or wrong by determining its relationship to a categorical imperative even without knowledge of the particular circumstances. Figure 2–3 provides a flow chart showing the processes of duty-oriented reasoning.

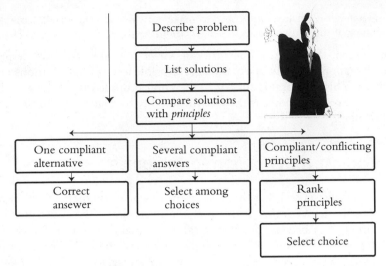

FIGURE 2–3 Duty-oriented Reasoning

Not long ago the media told of a family who could not find an acceptable bone marrow transplant donor for their daughter, who suffered from a rare form of cancer. In order to gain acceptable bone marrow they decided to have an additional child, hoping that the child would provide the match. Kantian theorists would find this action unacceptable, inasmuch as the baby was being used as a means rather than as an end of its own.

Criticisms of Kant

1. The exceptionless character of Kant's moral philosophy makes it too rigid for real life. Real-life situations are so varied that it is impossible to create rules that can guide us in all circumstances.
2. Morality cannot be derived from pure reason. The fact that we can feel pain and pleasure is central to morality. It is unlikely that we would care about morality if we did not feel pain or pleasure.
3. The disregard of the consequences of our actions can lead to disastrous results. We all have been hurt by well-meaning people who were overly concerned to "obey the law." It is often the spirit of the law, rather than the letter, that provides the arena for rational decisions. The Robert Bland proverb, "We may grasp virtue so hard that it becomes vicious," captures the essence of not considering the consequences of our decisions.
4. Even though nonhuman animals feel pain and pleasure, for Kant they do not have any independent moral standing since they are not rational beings.
5. It is possible to be faced with a conflict between two duties equally supported by an imperative. (The nurse who promises not to reveal that a patient has asked questions about euthanasia is asked by the family if the matter was discussed.)

Duty-oriented theorists obviously wish to promote a good result; however they feel that merely serving the good is not an adequate foundation for ethics. For these theorists the right action is one based upon a correct principle regardless of the results. For instance, if life is sacred, then murder is wrong, regardless of the circumstances leading to the act. Duty-oriented theorists argue among themselves as to how principles are derived, with some claiming the basis to be natural law, while others look to religious dictate, intuition, social contract, pure reason, or common sense.

One influential formulation of duty-oriented reasoning is the contract theory of John Rawls.[6] In this theory Rawls proposes that if a reasoning individual were placed in a social situation requiring a value choice without knowing what role they were playing in the situation (Rawls calls this the original position), the individual would chose the alternative that supported or favored the most disadvantaged person. This, then, becomes a restatement of the "golden rule," that when actions have an impact upon another, for these actions to be morally defensible, it must be the case that the actor would choose to be the recipient of an identical action by someone else under identical circumstances. The first principle of the social contract is to secure basic liberties for all individuals within the covenant:

> Each person possesses an inviolability founded on justice that even the welfare of the society as a whole cannot override. For this reason justice denies that the loss of freedom for some is made right by a greater good shared by others . . . the rights secured by justice are not subject to political bargaining or to the calculus of social interest.

Following this line of reasoning, the concern of an ethical society would be toward the care and support of its most disadvantaged citizenry, as they are the ones who are least able to speak for themselves. This is a decidedly duty-oriented position in that it establishes the duty of moral equality, which could not be bargained away regardless of social interest or the welfare of the society as a whole.

The individual whose intuitive moral sense leads him or her to believe that abortion is wrong under all circumstances, and the priest who maintains the confidentiality of the confessional even in the case of unreported incest, are both following the dictates of a duty-oriented or absolutist system. It is the exceptionless character of the duty-oriented position that gives most practitioners pause, as we seem always to be in situations of gray rather than black or white.

Neither theoretical position, consequence or duty oriented, has produced a theory that can be accepted under all circumstances. Both duty and consequence ethics pose grave problems in modern decision making. If we take, as an example, the question of the sanctity of life and an absolutist view prevails, modern medicine and technology might be placed on the side of saving every living individual from death regardless of intolerable costs, suffering of the family, or inability to restore life in a meaningful sense. Conversely, if a utilitarian view prevails, we might see arguments that would allow certain categories of handicapped individuals to be subjected to **euthanasia** on the basis that their removal served the best interest of society. Today, biomedical decision making is often based on an uneasy truce between the absolutist and consequentialist views, as practitioners seek a viable middle ground. In practice, rarely do you meet the individual who fails to consider the consequences of the situation, or one who is comfortable with decision making without reference to principles.

VIRTUE ETHICS

The lack of a convincing formulation for a duty-based or consequence-based ethical system that is able to overcome the major criticisms of each has, in the last two decades, led to an exploration of ethics, not understood as a set of rules to guide behavior, but as an attribute of character. Under this formulation, the first question is not "How do I act in this situation," but "How should I carry out my life if I am to live well?" The emphasis is taken off individual actions and the quandaries in which we find ourselves and put instead on what we can do to produce the sort of character that instinctively does the right thing. A good virtuous character is reflected in the display of such traits as courage, magnanimity, honesty, justice, temperance, and the like.

One result of the new trend has been to revisit the ethics of Aristotle. In his teachings, Aristotle distinguishes two kinds of virtue—intellectual and that of the character. Goodness of character was considered neither natural or unnatural, and it was thought to be produced by the practice of virtue. This practice created the habit of taking pleasure in virtuous acts, which then acted as a sign of a good life. Aristotle's traits of a virtuous character provided that:

1. Virtuous acts must be chosen for their own sake.
2. Choice must proceed from a firm and unchangeable character.
3. Virtue is a disposition to choose the mean.[7]

The virtuous person had a disposition of moderation toward the mean between two extremes. We all have experienced times when we needed to swing hard against the directions in which our passions were leading us. (Not every passion has a mean; for instance, there is no mean of murder, as murder is itself an extreme in interpersonal conduct.) Better examples can be found in courage, liberality, pride, ambition, good temper, truthfulness, shame, and justice.

Beyond character virtue, Aristotle also believed in intellectual virtues, such as practical wisdom. This he defined as the power of deliberation about things good for oneself. Neither practical wisdom nor character virtue could exist independently from each other.

A contemporary philosopher who has expanded Aristotle's work into a modern formulation of ethics is Alasdair MacIntyre.[8] MacIntyre holds that there have been many different conceptions of virtue that revolve around ideal characters associated with a variety of traditions. He isolates and describes several idealized characters such as Homeric (strength/warrior), New Testament (humility/slave), and Early American (industry/capitalist). Beyond these ideals, he believes in a core idea of virtue, of which courage, justice, and honesty are essential components.

In this ethical formulation, practices are the arena in which the virtues are exhibited, and it is only in terms of the particular practice that virtues can be defined. MacIntyre is thinking of social roles that provide standards of excellence and obedience to rules as well as common achievement goals toward some perceived good. To enter into the role of the physician, priest, or teacher is to enter into a practice, as well as to accept the authority of the standards of that role. In the example of the physician, once the individual accepts that practice, duty is determined by the role and the history of medical ethics. Figure 2–4 displays how decisions are made using virtue ethics reasoning.

In that practices have histories, the individual enters into a relationship not only with contemporary practitioners, but also with those who preceded us in the role. This is especially true of those who have come before us and have extended the practice to its present point. In this way, we learn from tradition, but tradition also learns from us. Our rapidly changing specialties do pose some problem for virtue ethics in that what may be considered a virtue in one period may be inappropriate in the next. The best example is perhaps nursing: The good practice in the 50s and 60s would have contained ample portions of virtues like submissiveness and respectfulness, whereas today these are being replaced with virtues such as patient advocate, patient teacher, etc. It is quite possible that on the same shift one could have several groups of nurses with differing views of what the "good nurse" is all about.

[handwritten margin note: These are roles not virtues.]

If we truly examine our actions as practitioners and look at what goes into our decision-making processes—in calculations of what is right or wrong in regard to professional duties—we would find we often are following the dictates of an idealized role. We are asking ourselves "What does the good nurse, physical therapist, or radiographer do when faced with this situation?" In this sense we are not calculating our duties from a teleological or deontological orientation, but are being guided by the duties imposed by our role and position in the health care team and society. One of the real problems with virtue ethics is that today's practitioners are being confronted by situations for which no role practices have been created, for which tradition provides no answers. An example of this new ground might be the

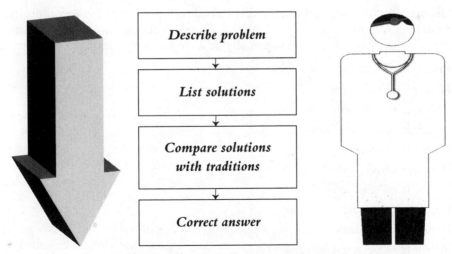

FIGURE 2–4 Virtue-oriented Reasoning

nurse or respiratory therapist in the position of not only disconnecting a ventilator from a patient in a persistent vegetative state, but also removing the feeding tube and IV lines.

Criticisms of Virtue Ethics

1. Virtue ethics generally does not provide specific directions in regard to decision making.
2. In that virtue ethics relies on traditional practices, it does not quickly respond to changes in the practice that require new sorts of moral responses.
3. The derivation of duty from one's social role is likely to lead to or perpetuate **classism**, sexism, etc.
4. A traditional emphasis makes **morality** depend on past experience rather than on reason. This environment provides little respect for creative solutions or personal autonomy.
5. Practitioners often find themselves attempting to address more than one set of idealized roles, which may come into conflict. (for example, the need to be a team player, and the need to be a whistle blower, in a case of negligent action).

SUMMARY

Over the course of our lives, each of us as humans develops a coherent set of attitudes, feelings, and opinions, with which we judge the world of actions around us—in terms of good and bad, right or wrong, positive or negative. This value system or world view is culturally shaped by the events of our lives and the traditions of our people.

Historically, philosophers and cultures have developed a list of value propositions that guide our views in regard to right and wrong. Although individual definitions might vary, the following would normally be included in a generalized value listing:

Principle of honesty

Principle of tolerance

Principle of lawfulness

Principle of truth telling

Principle of love

Principle of responsible behavior

Principle of benevolence

Principle of charity

Principle of equality

Principle of personal inviolability

Principle of justice

Several ethical systems have been proposed to assist and bring order to value-laden decision making. Clearly the settling of these issues by the flipping of a coin is unacceptable, as it would lead to an ethical pluralism, where any choice is as good as another. To allow a morally neutral society is not in keeping with social order and progress. Currently, the ethical systems with the highest level of acceptability are duty orientation, consequence orientation, and virtue ethics. Each of these systems allows for the examination of ethical problems and provides a framework for decision making. Each of these general systems with which we look at ethical problems has contemporary theorists with varying models, which can be classed as being duty, consequence, or virtue ethics oriented.

Each of the general ethical systems has been subjected to legitimate criticisms that they fail to overcome, and none at this point seems to have universal acceptance. When we examine our own personal value systems, we can be found to be duty oriented in some decisions, and consequentialistic in others. An individual could be very duty oriented in regard to an issue such as abortion, and yet approach the withdrawal or removal of life support from a consequence orientation. It has been noted that, just as in the fox hole there are no atheists, in the practice of health care, there is little comfort in decision making without a situational framework or the reliance on principle. Van Rensselaer Potter,[9] who is credited with coining the word "bioethics," explained that this new discipline had as its focus the traditional task of medical ethics, that of aiding the individual practitioner to make decisions and to live with them. Ethics, then, is a generic title that we give to systems that seek to bring sensitivity and method to the human task of decision making in the arena of moral values.

Whatever ethical framework one chooses in order to solve problems, usually the method will contain the six basic steps.

Step One—Identify the characteristics of the problem. Describe the problem and identify the principles involved. Who are the concerned parties? Who is charged with making the decision?

Step Two—Gather the facts of the case. What is fact, what is opinion? What are the legal ramifications? Has this issue been decided by the courts before? What documentation exists that outlines the problem?

Step Three—Examine the options with initial credibility. The more options you can think of, the more likely you are to find one you can support.

Step Four—Weigh and evaluate the potential options. What happens to the individuals involved, given each option? Has everyone been considered equally? "What principles are favored and which are sacrificed?" "What ethical system are you going to use to make the choice: utilitarianism, duty-oriented, or virtue ethics?

Step Five—Make your decision and act upon it.

Step Six—Assess and evaluate the results.

The next several chapters will-deal with health care issues and the methods used in coming to decisions. Within the clarification exercises, a variety of methods will be examined, but most will deal with the six basic steps as outlined.

CLARIFICATION EXERCISES

A. For this case, first justify your decision using duty-oriented reasoning and then follow using consequence-oriented reasoning.

As the local pharmacist, you have known the Smith family for years and consider them friends as well as customers and clients. Missy Smith has always been a favorite of yours and you have watched her grow into a very pretty thirteen-year-old. One day when no other customers are present, Missy asks you for a kit to test for pregnancy and pleads with you not to tell her family that she is sexually active.

B. Using the labels (cultural relativism, hedonism, consequence-oriented, virtue ethics and duty-oriented), identify the following statements:

    1. "If it feels good, do it."_____

    2. "Don't criticize until you walk a mile in their shoes."_____

    3. "The cost of maintaining the elderly on ventilators is beyond the cost the society can bear. After the age of 85, the elderly should not be placed on a ventilator, or should be taken off."_____

    4. "At the moment of conception a human comes into being, with all the rights and privileges of all other humans. In that life is sacred, nothing should be done that would sacrifice the fetus regardless of the situation."_____

    5. "As practitioners of the healing arts, we are to take care of the sick, even if they have conditions that threaten our personal health."_____

C. Virtue ethics depends upon an identifiable set of good practices. List some value-oriented acts that you are expected to assume as a practitioner of your specialty.

D. At the beginning of this chapter, we posed a series of everyday questions that involved value judgments. Answer each with a yes or no decision, and identify whether you arrived at your decision by duty-oriented, consequence-oriented, or virtue ethics reasoning. Use the models for decision making given in Figures 2–2, 2–3, and 2–4 to decide which line of reasoning you used.

    1. Is it right or wrong to take a gift from a patient?

    2. Is it acceptable to own a portion of a diagnostic clinic to which you refer patients?

    3. Should a pharmacist criticize a physician if the doctor will not change a drug order that is clearly not in the best interest of the patient?

    4. What is the nurse's duty when another nurse makes an error?

    5. Should you tell a patient who asks about the quality of specific medical care that in your opinion the physician is a jerk?

    6. As a radiographer you did a portable chest X ray on the wrong patient in Room 407. In that the patient is not coherent, and was not hurt by the process, do you have to report the error?

    7. As a physical therapist, if the patient could not afford the care but needed to continue therapy, would it be acceptable to falsify insurance papers in order to provide the appropriate care for your patient?

    8. As a respiratory therapist would it be acceptable to accept a finder's fee from a home health equipment company to which you referred your hospital patients?

    9. Would a surgical nurse with strong "pro-life" values be correct in refusing to take part in a therapeutic abortion?

REFERENCES AND SUGGESTED READING

1. Tom Beauchamp and Laurence McCullough, *Medical Ethics: The Moral Responsibilities of Physicians* (Englewood Cliffs, NJ: Prentice Hall, 1984), p. 37.
2. William Frankena, *Ethics* (Englewood Cliffs, NJ: Prentice Hall, 1973), pp. 87-88.
3. John Stuart Mill, *Utilitarianism, On Liberty,* and *Essay on Bentham,* ed. with intro. by Mary Warnock (New York: New American Library, 1974).
4. Joseph Fletcher, *Situation Ethics* (Philadelphia: Westminster Press, 1966).
5. Immanuel Kant, *Groundwork of the Metaphysic of Morals,*trans. J. J. Paton (New York: Harper and Row, 1964).
6. John Rawls, *A Theory of Justice* (Cambridge, MA: Harvard University Press, 1971).
7. Aristotle, *Nicomachean Ethics,* Trans. T. Irwin (Indianapolis, IN: Hackett Publishing Company, 1985).
8. MacIntyre, Alasdair. *After Virtue* (Notre Dame, IN: University of Indiana Press, 1981).
9. Van Rensselaer Potter, *Bioethics: Bridge to the Future* (Englewood, NJ: Prentice-Hall, 1973).

CHAPTER 3

Basic Principles of Health Care Ethics

Instructional Goal

The general goal of this chapter is to introduce the reader to the basic principles used in the analysis of moral dilemmas and to show how these principles function in health care delivery.

Instructional Objectives

At the end of this chapter the reader should understand and be able to:

1. Differentiate between morals and ethics.
2. Identify the basic principles involved in medical ethics, and show their application in our ethical codes.
3. Define the basic principles found in health care ethics.
4. Define paternalism and show how in the best sense it is a conflict between the principles of autonomy and beneficence.
5. Outline the nature of the special fiduciary relationship between the practitioner and the patient.
6. Differentiate between compensatory, retributive, procedural, and distributive justice.
7. Outline the ethical problem associated with side effects and the duty of nonmaleficence, and show how the principle of double effect is an attempt to resolve the issue.
8. Explain how the principle of "Informed Consent" is derived from the basic principle of autonomy.
9. Explain the types of cases where benevolent deception might be justified.

Glossary

Autonomy: Personal self-determination; the right of patients to participate in and finally decide questions involving their care.

Beneficence: The principle that imposes upon the practitioner to seek the good for the patient under all circumstances.

Benevolent Deception: The view that one can lie to the patient for his or her own good. It is the mechanism most often used when paternalism is advanced over patient autonomy.

Confidentiality: The principle that binds the practitioner to hold in strict confidence those things learned about a patient in the course of medical practice.

Ethics: A generic term that describes a variety of systems for providing rational analysis in regard to questions about the moral life.

Fiduciary Relationship: A special relationship of loyalty and responsibility that is formed between the patient and practitioner. The patient has the right to believe that the practitioner will maintain a higher level of accountability in regard to health care than that expected from most other relationships.

Informed Consent: In order for patients to be truly autonomous, they must understand the nature of the condition, the treatment options, and the risks involved. It is this information that forms the basis for informed consent.

Justice: The basic principle that deals with fairness, just deserts, and entitlements in the distribution of goods and services.

Nonmaleficence: The principle that imposes the duty to avoid or refrain from harming the patient. The practitioner who cannot bring about good for the patient is bound by duty to at least avoid harm.

Paternalism: The belief that one should, on the basis of doing good for the patient, limit the patient's personal autonomy. In the best sense it is a conflict between the basic principles autonomy and beneficence. What is to be done when patients choose not have the best done for them?

Placebos: Substances thought to be biologically inert that are given to patients so as to make them believe that they are getting medication. Although useful as a research practice, the clinical use of placebos creates real problems in the areas of patient autonomy, and the duty of truth telling.

Principle of Double Effect: A principle sometimes followed that is used to determine the morality of an act that has both beneficent and maleficent effects.

Role Fidelity: Each practice in health care has a prescribed role of practice. Role fidelity is the faithful practice of the duties contained in the particular practice. Role fidelity forms the basis for the ethical system known as virtue ethics.

Therapeutic Privilege: The right of the health care practitioner to provide care for patients without informed consent. Generally, these are rare cases in circumstances that involve emergency care, incompetent patients, or where sound medical judgment dictates that the truth would be a greater harm to the patient than the overcoming of his or her personal autonomy.

Veracity: Truth telling. The practice of health care is best served in a relationship of trust where practitioner and patient are bound to the truth.

APPLIED ETHICS

It appears to me that in Ethics, as in all other philosophical studies, the difficulties and disadvantages, of which history is full, are mainly due to a very simple cause: namely to the attempt to answer questions, without first discovering precisely what questions it is to which you desire an answer.

G. E. Moore, *Principia Ethica*, 1903

It is from our general world views that we have developed our societal morals and legal rights. These are in a continual state of evolution: As an illustration, society at one point in history will embrace slavery and then reject it, oppress women and disregard the handicapped and then struggle to create a legitimate space for all. These societal swings may come as reactions to such vague concepts as to "do good and avoid evil," or the "inherent dignity of the individual."

These concepts become part of the foundational fabric of our morals and ethics, and they undergo constant reinterpretation for every age and time. An excellent example of how certain values seem to capture the day and then fade to be replaced by others is the mid-19th-century slogan "Twin Relics of Barbarism: Slavery and Polygamy." Today this has little emotive impact, and yet in its time it justified the movement of armies. Likewise, the societal impact of "pro-choice" and "pro-life" arguments will eventually also run their course and seem to future generations as quaint as the twin relics.

To gain a clearer picture of the differences between morals and ethics, we might examine the distinction offered by the ethicist Joseph Fletcher,[1] who stated that "morality is what people believe to be right and good. . . . , while ethics is the critical reflections about morality and the rational analysis of it." **Ethics** then, is nothing more than a generic term for the study of how we make judgments in regard to right and wrong. Ethics offer a way of examining moral life.

Professional ethics, such as those found in medicine and law, are applied ethics designed to bring about the ethical conduct of the profession. In health care delivery, the major purpose might be the pursuit of health, with the prevention of death and the alleviation of suffering as secondary goals. The basic ethical principles that have been developed to allow health professionals to determine right and wrong in regard to value issues involving these goals are: autonomy, veracity, confidentiality, beneficence, nonmaleficence, justice, and role fidelity. Figure 3–1 illustrates a general hierarchy of thinking in regard to biomedical ethics, as we proceed from a general world view, to universal principles, to rules as found in our ethical codes, and finally to decisions. The universal principles have application for other areas of human endeavor such as politics, business, and the conduct of war.

The end good or major purpose of these various other pursuits will shift the focus from that given when the goal is health. This shifted focus can be seen in an incident taken from the World War II Battle for North Africa. The allies were faced with the dilemma of having two groups of soldiers needing antibiotics and only enough medication for one group. One group contained the traditional heroes, wounded in battle against the tank forces of the enemy, while the other group—perhaps equally traditional, but less heroic—had received their wounds in the local brothels, having

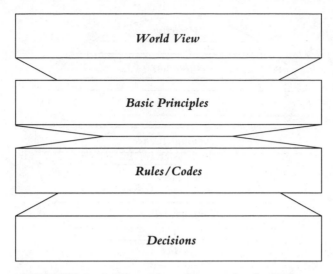

FIGURE 3–1 Hierarchy of Reasoning by Values

contracted venereal disease. Who should receive the limited antibiotics? If the choice had been purely medical, the decision might have been to treat the heroes wounded in battle, based on the severity of the wounds, or even by lottery to assure equality of access. However, inasmuch as the major factor became who could be made well quickly and returned to the battle line (a nonmedical focus), the easy decision was to treat those wounded in the brothels.

UNIVERSAL PRINCIPLES OF BIOMEDICAL ETHICS (Figure 3–2)

In the cases and problems that follow in later chapters, we will examine the focus that health care gives to the universal principles. It is from these principles that we derive the rules found in our professional codes of ethics. Although the principles are listed in a set order, it is not intended that they should be considered in any hierarchy of importance.

A. Autonomy. The word comes from the Greek *autos* (self) and *nomos* (governance). In health care, it has come to mean a form of personal liberty, where the individual is free to choose and implement one's own decisions, free from deceit, duress, constraint, or coercion. Three basic elements seem to be involved in the process: *the ability to decide*—for without adequate information, and intellectual competence, autonomy seems hollow; *the power to act upon your decisions*—it is obvious that those in the death camps of World War II could have make all the decisions they might have wished but lacked power to implement them; and finally *a respect for the individual autonomy of others*—it is the provision of a general respect for personal autonomy for both practitioner and patient alike that ennobles and professionalizes

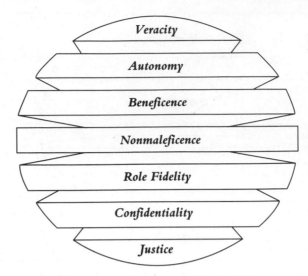

FIGURE 3–2 Universal Principles

the process. The term self-determination is often used synonymously with autonomy.

From the basic principle of autonomy, we have derived the rules involved in **"informed consent"** which generally contain the elements of disclosure, understanding, voluntariness, competence, and permission giving. It is obvious that the patient is not free to select an appropriate path if not given adequate information, stated in a manner that allows understanding. The information must be provided at a time when the patient is able to sort options rationally and is in a position to grant or refuse consent. Legal exceptions to the rules of informed consent under **therapeutic privilege** have been made in cases of emergency, incompetence, waiver, and when there is implied consent. A problematic area of therapeutic privilege is that of **benevolent deception**, where the practitioner is allowed to intentionally withhold information based on his or her "sound medical judgment" that to divulge the information might potentially harm the depressed and unstable patient.

One of the great areas of struggle in health care ethics is that of autonomy vs. paternalism. **Paternalism** is the intentional limitation of the autonomy of one person by another, where the person who limits autonomy appeals exclusively to grounds of benefit to the other person. Health care professionals have a special **fiduciary relationship** with patients based on the confidence placed in us and the inequality of our positions in regard to information. This relationship places an affirmative duty upon practitioners to seek the best for our patients. What, then, is to be done when the patient, acting on the impulse of personal autonomy, chooses a path away from health? Does the patient have the right to be wrong?

The American Hospital Association's Bill of Patient's Rights (Figure 3–3) states that "The patient has the right to refuse treatment to the extent permitted by law and to be informed of the medical consequences of his actions." This right in no way

AHA Policy   A Patient's Bill of Rights   **American Hospital Association**

This policy document presents the official position of the American Hospital Association as approved by the Board of Trustees and House of Delegates.

The American Hospital Association presents a Patient's Bill of Rights with the expectation that observance of these rights will contribute to more effective patient care and greater satisfaction for the patient, his physician, and the hospital organization. Further, the Association presents these rights in the expectation that they will be supported by the hospital on behalf of its patients, as an integral part of the healing process. It is recognized that a personal relationship between the physician and the patient is essential for the provision of proper medical care. The traditional physician-patient relationship takes on a new dimension when care is rendered within an organizational structure. Legal precedent has established that the institution itself also has a responsibility to the patient. It is in recognition of these factors that these rights are affirmed.

1. The patient has the right to considerate and respectful care.

2. The patient has the right to obtain from his physician complete current information concerning his diagnosis, treatment, and prognosis in terms the patient can be reasonably expected to understand. When it is not medically advisable to give such information to the patient, the information should be made available to an appropriate person in his behalf. He has the right to know, by name, the physician responsible for coordinating his care.

3. The patient has the right to receive from his physician information necessary to give informed consent prior to the start of any procedure and/or treatment. Except in emergencies, such information for informed consent should include but not necessarily be limited to the specific procedure and/or treatment, the medically significant risks involved, and the probable duration of incapacitation. Where medically significant alternatives for care or treatment exist, or when the patient requests information concerning medical alternatives, the patient has the right to such information. The patient also has the right to know the name of the person responsible for the procedures and/or treatment.

4. The patient has the right to refuse treatment to the extent permitted by law and to be informed of the medical consequences of his action.

5. The patient has the right to every consideration of his privacy concerning his own medical care program. Case discussion, consultation, examination, and treatment are confidential and should be conducted discreetly. Those not directly involved in his care must have the permission of the patient to be present.

6. The patient has the right to expect that all communications and records pertaining to his care should be treated as confidential.

7. The patient has the right to expect that within its capacity a hospital must make reasonable response to the request of a patient for services. The hospital must provide evaluation, service, and/or referral as indicated by the urgency of the case. When medically permissible, a patient may be transferred to another facility only after he has received complete information and explanation concerning the needs for and alternatives to such a transfer. The institution to which the patient is to be transferred must first have accepted the patient for transfer.

8. The patient has the right to obtain information as to any relationship of his hospital to other health care and educational institutions insofar as his care is concerned. The patient has the right to obtain information as to the existence of any professional relationships among individuals, by name, who are treating him.

9. The patient has the right to be advised if the hospital proposes to engage in or perform human experimentation affecting his care or treatment. The patient has the right to refuse to participate in such research projects.

10. The patient has the right to expect reasonable continuity of care. He has the right to know in advance what appointment times and physicians are available and where. The patient has the right to expect that the hospital will provide a mechanism whereby he is informed by his physician or a delegate of the physician of the patient's continuing health care requirements following discharge.

11. The patient has the right to examine and receive an explanation of his bill regardless of source of payment.

12. The patient has the right to know what hospital rules and regulations apply to his conduct as a patient.

No catalog of rights can guarantee for the patient the kind of treatment he has a right to expect. A hospital has many functions to perform, including the prevention and treatment of disease, the education of both health professionals and patients, and the conduct of clinical research. All these activities must be conducted with an overriding concern for the patient, and, above all, the recognition of his dignity as a human being. Success in achieving this recognition assures success in the defense of the rights of the patient.

FIGURE 3–3 A Patient's Bill of Rights *(Reprinted with permission of the American Hospital Association, copyright 1975.)*

speaks to the quality of the decisions, only to the patient's right to make them. As practitioners, we are fortunate to serve in professions that generally are viewed by our patients and clients as positions of confidence and trust. This allows most health care questions to be solved through a process of negotiation based on fidelity, respect, and shared values.

Complicating the process of autonomy are the cases in which it becomes necessary to limit autonomy because the patient could not be expected to comprehend sufficiently to make an authentic decision. For example, should a patient in severe pain be allowed to make a decision to refuse treatment based on the current pain, when the treatment will be lifesaving and restore normal function?

As our population continues to age, we have an ever-increasing number of individuals who are physically frail or who suffer from dementia. Even if we must, in the end, suspend some portion of their autonomy, who decides how much? The issue of autonomy and competency will be further discussed in Chapter 4.

B. Veracity. Veracity binds both the health practitioner and the patient in an association of truth. The patient must tell the truth in order that appropriate care can be provided. The practitioner needs to disclose factual information so that the patient can exercise personal autonomy.

The special fiduciary relationship that exists between patients and their health care practitioners is such that patients have the right to expect a higher level of truthfulness from us than others with whom they deal. If you were to buy a used car, you would hope that, in actual fact, the dealer would tell you the truth. If asked a direct question in regard to a specific problem, and the dealer lies, he is committing fraud; but in most jurisdictions he is not required to volunteer the information. The practitioner, however, is bound within the limitation imposed by her role to disclose all relevant information. The limitation imposed by role fidelity will be discussed in Chapter 12.

Even under the guise of benevolent deception, the idea of not telling the truth to patients is rather suspect. The suggestion is that the individual is not strong enough to tolerate the truth, or more time is needed to prepare the patient for an unpleasant fact. Unfortunately, this lack of truth telling leads to a slippery slope, for while it gives comfort to the one individual, it teaches all others involved—for example, family members, friends, housekeeping staff, and pink ladies—that health care practitioners lie to their patients. When these others become sick themselves, they remember the previous deception and feel they cannot rely on the word of the professionals. It would be a rare case that truly justified the lying to a patient. Modern health care is based on a complex set of covenants between the practitioner and patients, which work best under conditions of trust, veracity, and fidelity.

In his work, *The Death of Ivan Ilych*, Leo Tolstoy beautifully explains how benevolent deception forces the patient into the madness of playing a role unsuited to the circumstances:

> What tormented Ivan Ilych most was the deception, the lie, which for some reason they all accepted he was not dying but was simply ill . . . what tormented Ivan Ilych was that no one pitied him as he wished to be pitied. At certain moments after prolonged

suffering, he wished most of all (although he would have been ashamed to confess it) for someone to pity him as a sick child is pitied. He longed to be petted and comforted. . . .[2]

Medicine's attitude toward truth telling has always been in somewhat of an ambiguous place because of the way in which it can clash with the desire to do the best for the patient. The use of substances known as **placebos**, which the practitioner knows to be biomedically inert but which the patient feels are therapeutic, is a good example. Fundamental to the use of placebos is that the practitioner must engage in nondisclosure and deception in order for the practice to work. The defense offered is that the deception is used only for the welfare of the patient. This is a triumph of doing good (beneficence) over patient autonomy, which virtually forms the definition of paternalism. Figure 3-4 lists suggested rules to be considered and questions to be asked prior to participating in placebo therapy.[3]

Whereas it is conceivable that lying to the patient might become necessary to avoid some greater harm, it cannot be entered into lightly as it interferes directly with the person's autonomy. Tolerance for lying damages the system of health care delivery. Patients believe lies only because truthfulness is expected from health care providers. Once the patients begin to look for deceit, an essential element of good health care delivery will be lost.

In their work, *The Justification of Paternalism,* Gert and Sullivan[4] developed the following criteria to determine whether a paternalistic lie is justified:

1. The lie benefits the person lied to; that is, the lie prevents more evil than it causes for that particular person.

2. It must be possible to describe the greater good that occurs.

3. The individual should want to be lied to. If the evil avoided by the lie is greater than the evil caused by it, a person would be irrational not to want to be lied to.

- Placebos with active agents which may have harmful side effects are not acceptable.
- Placebos should not be given to patients without their consent.

? What is the condition being treated?
? What are the motives for the therapy?
? What is the placebo supposed to do?
? Are there alternatives that are less misleading?
? What is the patient/staff relationship?

FIGURE 3—4 Placebo Therapy Rules/Questions

4. Assuming equal circumstances, we would always be willing to allow the violation of veracity.

Allied health and nursing specialists should be committed to the truth. When faced with situations in which lying seems a rational solution, other alternatives must be sought. The harm to patient autonomy and the potential loss of practitioner credibility makes the lying to patients a practice that in almost all cases should be avoided.

C. Beneficence. The common English usage of the term beneficence suggests acts of mercy and charity, although it certainly may be expanded to include any action that benefits another. Most health care professions have statements that echo the *Hippocratic Oath* (Figure 3–5), which states that the physician will "apply measures for the benefit of the sick". The obligation to "help" imposes upon health care practitioners the duty to promote the health and welfare of the patient above other considerations, while attending and honoring their personal autonomy. In the pledge of the American Nurses' Association, this is clearly stated, "The nurse's

---

HIPPOCRATIC OATH

I swear by Apollo Physician and Asclepius and Hygieia and Panaceia and all the gods and goddesses, making them my witnesses, that I will fulfill according to my ability and judgment this oath and this covenant:

I will apply dietetic measures for the benefit of the sick according to my ability and judgment; I will keep them from harm and injustice.

I will neither give a deadly drug to anybody if asked for it, nor will I make a suggestion to this effect. Similarly I will not give to a woman an abortive remedy. In purity and holiness I will guard my life and my art.

I will not use the knife, not even on sufferers from stone, but will withdraw in favor of such men as are engaged in this work.

Whatever houses I may visit, I will come for the benefit of the sick, remaining free of all intentional injustices, of all mischief and in particular of sexual relations with both female and male persons, be they free or slaves.

What I may see or hear in the course of the treatment or even outside of the treatment in regard to the life of men, which on no account one must noise abroad, I will keep to myself holding such things shameful to be spoken about.

If I fulfill this oath and do not violate it, may it be granted to me to enjoy life and art, being honored with fame among all men for all time to come; if I transgress it and swear falsely, may the opposite of all this be my lot.

FIGURE 3–5

primary commitment is to the health, welfare, and safety of the client." The patients' assumption that the health care providers are struggling incessantly on their behalf is of great importance to their morale, especially for those who are summoning all their strength to fight illness.

In an earlier age, when medical science had less to offer, the duty of beneficence was rather straightforward. Prior to this century, even after exhausting all efforts to help, health care providers were often only able to sit by the bed dispensing good psychological support, unable to arrest the disease process. However, with advanced life-support techniques, it is possible and common today to arrest the process of death, but at the same time to fail in the restoration of life in a human sense, the life captured in events, life in a biographical sense. Life without awareness, without relationships, is perhaps not a beneficence but an additional form of injury.

Questions arise: Is the restoration of life that appears to have no value to the individual, beneficence? Are the staggering fiscal and emotional costs justifiable? When does the effort cease to be beneficent? With modern medicine, where technology often overwhelms resources, it has become necessary to use cost/benefit ratio analysis to determine where beneficence ends and maleficence (doing harm) begins. In an earlier time, prior to antibiotics, pneumonia was known as "an old man's friend," as it was commonly the illness that ended life filled with pain and suffering. In Chapters 7 and 8 we will discuss the issues of withholding and withdrawing life support as well as the current controversy involving active euthanasia.

D. Nonmaleficence. Most health care professional pledges or codes of care echo the principle paraphrased from the Hippocratic Oath statement "I will never use treatment to injure or wrong the sick." In some way, this seems very similar to the duty of beneficence, where the practitioner works to maximize the good for the patient and to minimize harm. T. Beauchamp and J. Childress[5] distinguish the principles in the following way:

Nonmaleficence

1. One ought not to inflict evil or harm

Beneficence

2. One ought to prevent evil or harm
3. One ought to remove evil or harm
4. One ought to do or promote good

All the statements of beneficence involved positive action toward preventing, or removing harm, and promoting the good. In the nonmaleficence statement, the admonition is stated in the negative, to refrain from inflicting harm.

The technology of modern health care and therapeutics has made this a most difficult principle to follow, because much of what we do has unfortunate secondary or side effects. For example, when steroids are administered to the asthmatic patient to relax the smooth muscles of the airway, often the side effect of Cushings Syndrome occurs. Some of the newer antibiotics given to fight infections have

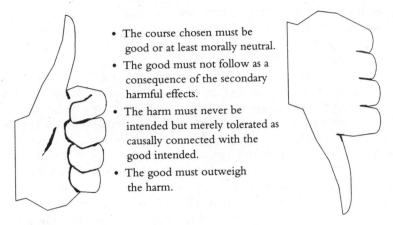

- The course chosen must be good or at least morally neutral.
- The good must not follow as a consequence of the secondary harmful effects.
- The harm must never be intended but merely tolerated as causally connected with the good intended.
- The good must outweigh the harm.

FIGURE 3—6 Principle of Double Effect (Guiding Elements)

ototoxicity and nephrotoxicity as side effects. Analgesics such as morphine given for pain may lead to a suppression of respiration. In attempting to maintain the ethical position of nonmaleficence in these cases, some practitioners have explained their actions through the **principle of double effect.**[6] With this concept the secondary effects may be foreseen, but can never be the intended outcomes. The practitioner could, when necessary, ethically prescribe or administer morphine for pain, while understanding that the analgesic suppresses respiration—so long as the intended effect is the former and never the latter and the good intentions equal or outweigh harmful effects. The elements contained within the principle of double effect are outlined in Figure 3–6. Although intuitively persuasive and described and defended in many duty-oriented works, the principle of double effect has detractors who feel that unwanted effects of actions that are foreseen and still allowed within the course of treatment become intended effects. Even if the principle of double effect is finally put to rest and found not to be a useful formulation for practice, it still asks the right question: Under what circumstances can one be said to act morally when some of the manifold foreseeable effects of that action are harmful? Figure 3-7 points out how the basic principles are considered almost common sense and intuitively correct.

E. Confidentiality. The American Hospital Association's Patient's Bill of Rights rules 5 and 6 outline the individual's right to privacy in health care:

5. The patient has the right to every consideration of his privacy concerning his own medical care program. Case discussion, consultation, examination, and treatment are confidential and should be conducted discreetly. Those not directly involved in his care must have permission of the patient to be present.

6. The patient has the right to expect that all communications and records pertaining to his care should be treated as confidential.

Confidentiality is an important aspect of the trust that patients place in health care professionals. If the patient felt that information in regard to his or her body or

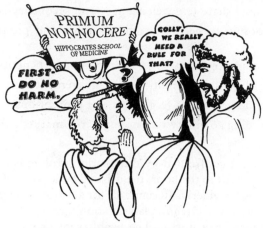

FIGURE 3–7

condition was the subject of public conversation used to brighten the coffee break in the cafeteria, or was subject to release to publications, a great barrier between practitioner and patient would exist. This fear of disclosure has, in the past, led minors with sexually transmitted diseases to suffer without care rather than to seek aid, knowing that the system required the health care system to notify their parents.

With the advent of computer technology and sophisticated information systems, personal confidentiality is beset in all aspects of our lives. This is especially true with medical information systems where patient information can be brought up on a CRT screen in a variety of areas throughout the hospital, making this information available to all who are on the system.

In a survey that looked at the expectations of patients, medical students, and house staff in regard to the issue of confidentiality, it was found that patients expected a more rigorous standard of confidentiality than that in current practice [7]. In the study, house staff and medical students indicated that they frequently discussed patients with spouses and informally with each other at parties. While current practice may require that cases be discussed in professional settings to gather other opinions, great care must be taken to warrant the confidence that is placed in us by our patients. The breaching of confidentiality has serious implications. It threatens to harm our patients, our professions, and the society in general that depends upon the services we provide.

F. Justice. The maintenance of this ethical principle is seemingly very simple in the abstract and complex in application, as it looks at the concepts of fairness, just deserts, and entitlements. What is due to an individual? In a just society, we require procedural justice or due process in cases of disputes between individuals. In health care we deal with *distributive justice* as we struggle with the distribution of scarce resources. Perhaps the most famous formulation is that stated by Aristotle that "equals must be treated equally and un-equals must be treated unequally."

In our society we use several methods for the distribution of goods and services, attempting in some measure to provide a system in which individuals receive their due share:[8]

1. To each, an equal share (e.g., elementary and secondary education)
2. To each, according to need (e.g., aid to needy and programs such as food stamps)
3. To each, according to effort (e.g., unemployment benefits)
4. To each, according to contribution (e.g., retirement systems)
5. To each, according to merit (e.g., jobs and promotions)
6. To each, according to ability to pay (e.g., free market exchange)

In health care we are confronted by distribution problems that seem to provide better care to the rich than to the poor, the urban dweller over the rural, the middle-aged over the child or the elderly. Recent calls for a national health system much like that found in Canada, or the Oregon plan to ration care, can be seen as an attempt to better apply the principle of justice. The problem of providing for fair and equal distribution of health care would be difficult even if we assumed a world of unlimited resources. Once we factor in problems of scarcity, practitioner self-determination, maldistribution of resources, and costs, it becomes overwhelming.

A further discussion of the principle of justice will follow in Chapter 11. Complicating the issue of just distribution is a lack of agreement upon what constitutes health. Certain groups, such as the World Health Organization (WHO), define it in the broadest terms: "a state of complete physical, mental, and social well-being, and not merely the absence of infirmity."[9] In that this definition somewhat guarantees everything for everybody, it becomes hard to imagine the distribution system that could accommodate such promises.

Another interesting aspect is the area of compensatory justice, where individuals seek compensation for a wrong that has been done. This has become a far more important aspect of medicine in light of the cases such as those where harm was caused by asbestos and other materials placed in our bodies and environment. Recent cases where cigarette smokers have attempted to receive compensation from tobacco companies for their lung cancer or emphysema suggest how large an issue this may become in the future.

Similar to compensatory justice is the ancient call for retributive justice or "an eye for an eye and a tooth for a tooth." Unlike compensatory justice, where fines and compensation for injury are requested, retributive justice calls for equal suffering. Given the power of the argument (usually heard first from our mothers) that "two wrongs never make a right," retribution may have very little to do with any form of behavior suitable for the health care arena.

G. Role Fidelity. Modern health care is the practice of a team, as no single individual can maintain the data bank of information needed to provide rational care. Contained within the designation of allied health are over 100 individual professions, which in combination with nursing provide over 80 percent of our national health care. The nature of these specialties shapes the way in which the individual practitioner will respond to basic questions of biomedical ethics. An example of this might be the duty of the respiratory care practitioner not to tell a patient's family how critical the situation is, while the attending physician might have an obligation to relate the information. Whatever the assigned role, the ethics of health care require that the practitioner practice faithfully within the constraints of the role. Most often the areas of acceptable practice are contained and prescribed by the scope of practice of the state legislation that enables that profession's practice.

SUMMARY

In general, morality is concerned with what people believe to be right and good conduct. It is transmitted from generation to generation, evolving and being reinterpreted for each age. This broad understanding of what is right and wrong in human conduct is taught to us by our families, religion, national culture, and legal structure.

Ethics is that part of philosophy that deals with systematic approaches to questions of morality. It provides the intellectual framework that allows us to analyze and make decisions in regard to moral choices. In no area of our lives are we more pressed by value-laden decisions than that of health care. The enormous power gained by our scientific successes raises questions that have never previously been posed, such as:

Should the elderly be provided the same level of health care as that provided for children?

Should patients with orders "Do Not Resuscitate" orders be treated in intensive care?

Must a health care provider who is HIV positive relate this to patients?

Who should live when not all can live?

Is there a morality to mercy killing?

Can health care practitioners work for the patient and be socially responsible for cost containment at the same time?

What constitutes life? What is a person?

Is there a right to health care? If there is a right, what is the limit of that right?

Is there a moral difference between removing a ventilator from a patient, and removing IV tubes and a nasal gastric tube?

What is the meaning of confidentiality when, on the average, over 75 different individuals have access to information from our medical records?

Who shall be denied lifesaving treatment when there is not enough for all?

The increased usage of high technology, the breakthroughs in scientific research, the adoption of team medicine, and the easy access to data have rapidly brought major changes to the delivery of health care and have created a host of new moral dilemmas for which there are no easy solutions. However, answers must be found because the very concept of value-free medicine is unworkable, and because health care practitioners are forced into the process of making choices with which we as individuals and a society can live.

All forms of professional ethics draw from the same well of basic principles that shape our concepts of right and wrong in all aspects of our lives. The nature of our profession, however, and it's basic purposes and goals will give these basic principles a unique focus. Therefore decision-making analysis from a legal, military, or health care perspective will often bring out decidedly different views of what is right in a given situation. Even within the different specialties of health care, the requirements of role duty will shape the analysis of ethical problems. In recent times, many questions involving health care ethics have been litigated in the courts for final decisions. The nature of these decisions do not always flow from ethically correct precepts. Something truly can be socially correct, medically possible, and legally permissible—and yet be morally reprehensible for the individuals involved.

In general, the basic principles involved in health care ethics are: Autonomy, veracity, beneficence, nonmaleficence, justice, confidentiality, and role fidelity. Often decision making in health care takes the form of an appeal for justification, based on an attempt to be true to one of these basic principles.

Professional codes of ethics can be seen as rules derived from the universal principles to bring about the goals of the profession. Although drawing from the same universal principles, they are shaped by the needs of the specific profession. An example of this is the clinical laboratory science focus on the need for detail and exactness. The respiratory care practitioners might find a focus in being directed by physicians and staying within the scope of practice. The code of ethics for medical record personnel stresses the duty of confidentiality.

CLARIFICATION EXERCISES

A. For the following code of ethics, identify the universal principle that is being addressed with each rule. For example, a rule that requires a nurse not to disclose personal information would be addressing the universal principle of confidentiality

A.N.A. Code for Nurses

1. The nurse provides services with respect for human dignity and the uniqueness of the client unrestricted by considerations of social or economic status, personal attributes, or the nature of health problems.
   Principle(s) involved_____

2. The nurse safeguards the client's right to privacy by judiciously protecting information of a confidential nature.
   Principle(s) involved_____

3. The nurse acts to safeguard the client and the public when health care and safety are affected by the incompetent, unethical, or illegal practice of any person.
   Principle(s) involved_____

4. The nurse assumes responsibility and accountability for individual nursing judgments and actions.
   Principle(s) involved_____

5. The nurse maintains competence in nursing.
   Principle(s) involved_____

6. The nurse exercises informed judgment and uses individual competence and qualifications as criteria in seeking consultation, accepting responsibilities, and delegating nursing activities to others.
   Principle(s) involved_____

7. The nurse participates in activities that contribute to the ongoing development of the profession's body of knowledge.

    Principle(s) involved_____

8. The nurse participates in the profession's efforts to implement and improve standards of nursing.

    Principle(s) involved_____

9. The nurse participates in the profession's efforts to protect the public from misinformation and misrepresentation and to maintain the integrity of nursing.

    Principle(s) involved_____

10. The nurse participates in the profession's efforts to establish and maintain conditions of employment conducive to high-quality nursing care.

    Principle(s) involved_____

11. The nurse collaborates with members of the health professions and other citizens in promoting community and national efforts to meet the health needs of the public.

    Principle(s) involved_____

B. Review the code of ethics for your specialty to determine what basic principle is being addressed with each rule. (The codes of ethics for the following specialties are found in Appendix A: Nursing, Medical Technology, Pharmacy, Respiratory Care, Physicians, Radiographers, Medical Record Specialists, Physical Therapists, and Occupational Therapists)

C. Does the code of ethics for your specialty have a rule that addresses each of the basic principles (autonomy, veracity, beneficence, nonmaleficence, justice, confidentiality and role fidelity)?

D. Compare your code to the one for the American Medical Association. In what way does yours differ? In what way does your code reflect the nature of your specialty?

E. In the following cases, identify the principle(s) involved and state a rule from your specialty code of ethics that might be used to address the issue.

1. In a voluntary outpatient psychiatric clinic in California, a young man disclosed to his psychologist that he intended to kill a young woman. From previous conversations, the psychologist knew the identity of the woman and became very concerned. After the young man had left his office, the psychologist consulted with his superior and they decided to have the man stopped by the security person at the gate.

    When security stopped the man as he was leaving the clinic, they became concerned about his legal rights in that he appeared to them to be rational and to threaten no danger to himself or others. They related this information to the psychiatrist on duty, who then decided to allow the man to leave and ordered the records of the event destroyed.

    The young man then proceeded to carry out his intentions and shortly thereafter took the life of the young woman. The parents of the woman, upon finding out about what had occurred, sued the clinic.

    The clinic staff defended their actions on the basis that (1) many individuals fantasize about doing harm to others without carrying out the threat, and (2) to repeat the information gathered during therapy would bring them into an ethical problem of breaching confidentiality. They held that if the patients did not have faith that what they said during therapy was going to be held in confidence, in actual fact they would not continue to reveal anything of significance.

    Principle(s) involved_____

    In your specialty code of ethics, which rule might have application?

    What is your own personal decision concerning the lawsuit in this case?

2. You and Joseph Bradshaw have been friends and colleagues for some time. You are graduates from the same physical therapy program and now work at the same

rehabilitation center. This has been a hard year for Joseph, as he has just come through a very difficult divorce, and you have attempted to befriend him. Recently you have noticed that he has been acting a bit strange, laughing at inappropriate times and having mood swings—between being very quiet to talking a mile a minute. You suspect that your friend has begun to abuse drugs.

Your suspicions are confirmed one day in a conversation, in which he reveals to you that he has had a hard time sleeping of late, and is taking pills to help him sleep and then other pills to keep him going through the day. Joseph asks you to keep his problem a secret, as he is sure that this is just something that he will need to work out as he gets over his divorce.

The next day during morning review of the patients, Joseph seems to be falling asleep during report. Later your department head, who knows of your friendship with Joseph, approaches you and asks, "What is the matter with Joe?" You wonder what to say.

Principle(s) involved_____

What rule in your specialty code of ethics might have application in this case?

Before you come to a personal decision, first list all the options that have some credibility. After you have developed your options list, then estimate how each of the parties involved will fair under each of the options.

F. In Greek literature there are several models for health care practice. Two with significance for our time are the cult of Aesculapius, and the cult of Hygeia.

The cult of Aesculapius is strictly a patient/health care practitioner affair aimed at the getting the particular individual physically well. In this light, care would be aggressively patient centered, and the practitioner would not mix social, political, or economic considerations with the care of the patient.

The cult of Hygeia (daughter of Aesculapius) uses the broader social or public health model of prevention as well as therapy as the context for care. The term hygiene means "good for health." This approach is based on the prevention of disease rather than treatment. Hygeia is the public health or public interest way of looking at health care delivery.

Examine the American health care delivery system, and indicate which of the models best fit what we are currently doing in our culture.

Examine the particular practice of your specialty. Which of the Greek models is it most closely aligned with Aesculapius, or Hygeia?

G. Are there basic ethical principles missing from your professional code of ethics? If so, write rules that should be added to your code to address these areas.

H. A case often cited that looks at the principle of veracity is that of the husband and wife who are both in a nursing home. The husband has a heart attack and the wife is brought from another floor. Before she can get to the room the man dies, but to spare the woman pain, the staff allows her to think that he is still alive when she gets to the room. In that she is frail and feeble, with poor eyesight, she does not know that he is dead. The woman is then told that her husband's respiration is growing weaker and that he appeared to have been waiting for her before he died. As she leaves the room, she tells the staff that she is so glad that he waited for her so that she could see him alive one more time.

Using the Gert and Sullivan criteria listed in the chapter under the principle of veracity, does the above case justify the lying? Explain your answer.

REFERENCES AND SUGGESTED READINGS

1. Joseph Fletcher, *The Ethics of Genetic Control* (Garden City, New York: Anchor Books, 1974) p. xiii.
2. Leo Tolstoy, *The Death of Ivan Illych and Other Stories* (New York: New American Library, 1960).

3. Marilyn Desmarais, "The Nurse's Ethical Guide to Placebo Giving," *California Nurse,* May 1988.
4. Bernard Gert and Charles Culver, "The Justification of Paternalism," in *Medical Responsibility* ed. W. Robinson, and M. Pritchard (Clifton, NJ: The Humana Press, 1979) pp. 1–9.
5. Tom Beauchamp and James Childress, *Principles of Biomedical Ethics* (New York: Oxford University Press, 1989), p. 119.
6. Robert Walker, "DNR in the OR," *Journal of the American Medical Association* 266, no. 17 (November 1991): 2407–2411.
7. Barry Weiss, "Confidentiality Expectations of Patients, Physicians, and Medical Students," *Journal of the American Medical Association* 247 (1982): 2695–97.
8. Gene Outka, "Social Justice and Equal Access to Health Care," in *Ethics and Health Policy,* ed. R. M. Veatch and R. Branson (Cambridge: Ballinger Publishing Co., 1976).
9. *Preamble* to the Constitution of the World Health Organization, adopted 1946.

CHAPTER 4

Autonomy vs. Paternalism: A Contest Between Virtues

Instructional Goal

The general goal of this chapter is to outline the nature of the conflict between autonomy and paternalism, and to discuss the requirements and elements of informed consent. A secondary goal will be to investigate the nature of competency determination.

Instructional Objectives

At the end of this chapter the reader should understand and be able to:

1. Define paternalism.
2. Describe how paternalism is, in its best sense, a result of physician beneficence.
3. List and describe the four models of physician/patient interaction as outlined by Robert Veatch. Explain why the contractual model seems best suited for today's practice.
4. Define and list the elements of informed consent.
5. Differentiate between the professional community standard and the reasonable patient standard, and explain how the latter better serves the needs of the autonomous patient.
6. Explain why a more subjective standard than the professional community standard or the reasonable patient standard may be needed to protect patient autonomy.

7. Define therapeutic privilege, list the situations where it is used, and explain the problems of benevolent deception.

8. List several groups in our society that would have limited autonomy.

9. Outline the major elements of competency determination.

10. Explain how the First Amendment of the Constitution protects the autonomy of religious individuals who have beliefs that conflict with current medical practice.

Glossary

Abandoned: Once a patient/practitioner relationship is established, the health care services must continue or the practitioner may face the legal action of abandonment. The relationship may be discontinued only under very specific circumstances.

Ad litim: A guardian ad litem is a person given the power and duty to act in behalf of another, for example, a legally incapacitated person for purposes of a lawsuit.

Authentic Decision: An authentic decision is one that is in keeping with the individual's past choices and known preferences.

Competency: Having the ability to make sound authentic judgments for oneself. Usually this means that the patient is able to understand the nature of the condition, the options available, and the risks involved.

Patient-Centered Standard: A standard holding that the information needed is that required by the individual to make a rational judgment. This would be a very subjective standard, given that some patients may not meet the criteria of a hypothetical reasonable person.

Professional Autonomy: Once a patient/health care professional relationship is established, the practitioner has a duty to provide care but is not obliged to perform services that he or she finds morally repugnant. Health care providers may, under such circumstances, withdraw from their obligations to provide services.

Professional Community Standard: A standard stating that the amount of care or amount of disclosure provided should be judged appropriate if it is equal to that provided by other practitioners in the local community.

Reasonable Patient Standard: A standard that holds that the physician must provide enough information to the patient so that a *hypothetical* reasonable person could understand and make autonomous decisions.

VALUE PREFERENCE AS THE BASIS OF HEALTH CARE DECISIONS

The objection of some of the laymen concerned about the problem has been to what they call the "Father Knows Best" authoritative, paternalistic attitude of physicians. In fact, if "Father" didn't know best, he ought to retire from the case.

Noted Surgeon

If the health care practitioner is the expert and if health is a universal good, it would seem that the patient, who is a stranger to this specialized world of medicine, would just lie there and allow the medical team to work on his or her behalf. The problem with this reasoning lies in the fact that, although health is a universal good, it is not the only one. The good life, however we define it, contains many goals beyond health—which, at times, have a higher personal value. A hypothetical case that looks at how a variety of factors interplay to shape decisions is that of an author who contracts a terminal disease. His physician knows of a drug that, if taken, will extend the author's life by ten years. Without the medicine, the prognosis is two to three years. Following the physician's recommendation, the author takes the medication and starts what he anticipates will be his greatest work. Unfortunately, the medication leaves his mind clouded, and he loses his creative ability to write. He is faced with the problem of taking the medication and extending his life to ten rather cloudy, noncreative years or not taking the drug and shortening his life by seven or eight years. Without the drug, however, during his remaining two to three years he would be clear minded, which would potentially allow him to finish his greatest work.

In this hypothetical case, the author discontinues the treatment against his doctor's recommendations. The desire to complete what he considered to be his greatest literary accomplishment had a higher personal value than did an extended nonproductive life. The example shows that health care decisions are matters not only of medical expertise, but also of individual value preferences.

From Paternalism to Patient Autonomy

An irony of health care is that, in an earlier age, when practitioners had less to offer by way of scientific evidence for their cures and nostrums, society allowed them a greater role in medical decision making. Now, when every treatment is subjected to scientific method and scrutiny, the patient is demanding and receiving a greater role in the decision-making process. The scope of the distance we have come in this process from physician paternalism to patient autonomy can be seen from two excerpts—one from the *Code of Ethics of the American Medical Association* (1848) and the other from the American Hospital Association's *A Patient's Bill of Rights*.

1848 Code, Section 6.

The obedience of a patient to the prescriptions of his physician should be prompt and implicit. He should never permit his own crude opinions. . . .[1]

Patient's Bill of Rights.

4. The patient has the right to refuse treatment to the extent permitted by law and to be informed of the medical consequences of his action.[2]

Health care practitioners down through the ages have prescribed faith and obedience as essential aspects of the cure. Roughly speaking, *paternalism* consists of acting in a way that is believed to protect and advance the interests of another even through the actions may be against the desires, or may in the fact limit the freedom of action, of the individual. At it's best, paternalism comes into being when the desire to honor the principle of beneficence comes into conflict with the patient's autonomy.

AUTONOMY VS. BENEFICENCE

The most eloquent statement and defense for personal autonomy is found in the essay *On Liberty* by John Stuart Mill. In this work, the author holds that the only purpose for which power can be rightfully exercised over any other member of a civilized community against his will is to prevent harm to others.

> His own good, either physical or moral, is not a sufficient warrant. He cannot be compelled to do or forebear because it will be better for him to do so, because it will make him happier, because, in the opinion, to do so would be wise or even right. These are good reasons for remonstrating with him, but not for compelling him or visiting him with any evil in case he does otherwise.[3]

The issue is more complex than who is in charge or even who knows best. The real issue is which of the basic ethical principles holds supremacy in a given situation. Should it be the personal liberty of self-determination under the principle of autonomy even at the expense of forcing the health care provider to do less than could be done, or should it be under the principle of practitioner beneficence, where care is provided even in cases where the patient wishes to be left alone?

Should alert, rational patients be allowed to refuse reasonable care if that decision sacrifices their lives or health? A secondary question is, "What duty do health care providers have in this choice?" Can the practitioner assist after the patient has made a decision that is medically incorrect and, if followed, would lead to personal harm?

What of the practitioner's **professional autonomy**? Can a patient's desire to be treated in a particular way overcome the autonomy of the health care provider? For instance, if a patient demands an abortion from a physician with a pro-life view, whose autonomy should prevail? In general, the practitioner is not required to act contrary to basic personal values and beliefs. However, if a patient/provider relationship has been established, and the practitioner feels that he or she must withdraw services, care must be taken to assure that the patient is not **abandoned** and is referred appropriately.

The attitudes of some practitioners toward patient autonomy can be brought into focus by considering what is meant when we say "Mr. Jones is a good patient," or "Physicians and nurses do not make good patients." Often what is meant is that Mr. Jones follows orders but that physicians and nurses are assertive and noncompliant. In this light, "good" indicates an individual who allows the medical staff to make all the decisions. In his essay "What Does the Word Good Mean in Good Patient," Pedro lain Entralgo outlined several requirements for the sick person vis-à-vis the physician. In this outline, the emphasis is clearly on the side of compliance rather than self-determination.[4]

1. The sick person is reasonably obedient, but not absolutely submissive. By obeying his doctor, the sick person should not cease to be a free human being, a person. A slave's obedience is not the best kind for being a good patient in times of illness.

2. The sick person opens himself truthfully to his physician. Whether his confidence in whomever treats him is great or small, the sick person owes his doctor the truth about himself as soon as the doctor asks. Even when he confides little to his physician, the sick person can and ought to be a good patient.

The arguments for and against paternalism have led to disagreements in regard to when practitioner beneficence can validly overcome a patient's autonomous action. Can the physician, under the guise of doing good, force a patient to receive lifesaving care, even against his or her will? Children and the elderly often find their autonomy limited in that they are held to be incompetent and incapable of assessing risk to themselves.

PROVIDER/PATIENT RELATIONSHIP

Robert Veatch proposed a series of hypothetical models used for the examination of the physician/patient relationship. In these models the relationships take four basic forms:[5]

Engineering Model

In this pattern, the physician acts as a scientist who deals only with facts. The physician gathers the information, explains the material to the patient, and then divorces himself from the decision. The physician allows the patient to make the decision and follows the dictates of this choice. Although this model allows for a high level of patient autonomy, it permits no professional determinism. The practitioner would not be allowed to exercise personal values, and if called upon would perform duties that might possibly be personally abhorrent.

Priest Model

This is a highly paternalistic model, where the physician operates from the moral position of knowing what is best for the patient. It often takes the form of "As your physician I recommend . . . ." The patient is led to believe that his or her opinion is not of the same value as that of the learned physician. This form of paternalism goes well beyond paternalism based on the concept of beneficence, and is more a matter of personal control.

Collegial Model

This model suggests that the physician and patient should see themselves as colleagues solving the common problem of eliminating illness. Mutual trust and confidence drive the model as the two work toward the shared and common goal in a collegial, harmonious, atmosphere of equality. While this model may have some element of reality in the radical health movement, or in free clinics, it has limited usage in other medical arenas.

Unfortunately, due to ethnic, class, social, and/or value differences between patients and their physicians, a collegial atmosphere of equality is more a pipe dream than a reality. The physician as our pal is not a picture that most of us hold for any period of time.

Contractual Model

This is a shared decision-making model where the patient is accorded the right to make decisions and to have control over his own life whenever significant decisions are to be made. Once the highly value-laden decisions are made, the patient relies on the technical experience and skills of the medical team for most of the decisions in regard to care. Both the physician and patient have the option to reopen the contract and to leave the relationship if the decisions of one run contrary to the value systems or are abhorrent to the other. The contractual model allows both individuals to interact in an atmosphere of both obligations and expected benefits.

INFORMED CONSENT

It is from the struggle between paternalism and autonomy that the basis for the doctrine of informed consent has been derived. This moral and legal doctrine is a product of the last half of the twentieth century as judges have sought to protect the patient's right to greater freedom of choice. Informed consent binds the physician to an adequate disclosure and explanation of the treatment and the various options and consequences. Simply stated, informed consent requires that before any risky or invasive procedures can be performed, the health care practitioner must inform the patient of pertinent details about the nature of the procedure, its purpose, potential risks involved, and any reasonable alternatives that might be chosen. Figure 4–1 lists the elements of informed consent found in most definitions.

---

1. Disclosure: The nature of the condition, the various options, potential risks, the professional's recommendation, and the nature of consent as an act of authorization.

2. Understanding: In the United States, most states require that the physician provide information at a level that a *hypothetical* reasonable patient would understand.

3. Voluntariness: No efforts toward coercion, manipulation, or constraint are allowed. The patient must be in a position to practice self-determination.

4. Competence: Decisions in regard to competence usually take into account experience, maturity, responsibility, and independence of judgment.

5. Consent: An autonomous authorization of the medical intervention.

FIGURE 4–1 Elements of Informed Consent

STANDARDS OF DISCLOSURE

It is informed consent that allows autonomous self-determination. The main struggle in the courts has been to determine what standards should govern the level of disclosure. Two standards have been proposed, the **Professional Community Standard** and the **Reasonable Patient Standard.**[6]

Professional Community Standard

The health care provider is bound to provide the amount of information that would be expected from other reasonable practitioners within the community in similar situations. This formed the basis of the decision in the 1906 *Natanson v. Kline* case,[7] which set forth what a physician must disclose in regard to the side effects of cobalt therapy. This standard was based on the concept that the practitioner and patient were bound in a special fiduciary relationship in which the difference in levels of information and patient trust binds the professional to act in the patient's behalf without allowing any conflict of interest. The amount of information provided and the nature of the information would be determined by the traditions of the practice and the professional community. The application of this standard seems to generate a great number of problems, since the focus is not on patient understanding but rather on the physician's standard of practice. Since there is often a wide gap between the social, economic, and educational level of the physicians and their patients, even given the best of intentions this standard does not necessarily lead to a level of communication that allows for true patient autonomy.

Reasonable Patient Standard

This holds that the amount and kind of information needed is that which a hypothetical reasonable person would need in order to understand the nature of the condition and the various options. This standard was articulated in the 1972 *Canterbury v. Spence* case,[8] where the court ruled that "True consent to what happens to one's self is the informed exercise of a choice, and that entails an opportunity to evaluate knowledgeably the options available and the risks attendant upon each." The rationale for this standard is that the type and amount of information needed must be at the patient's level if he or she is truly to be autonomous as a decision maker. One criticism of the reasonable patient standard is the nature of the "hypothetical person": Who is to say that this person is anything like the patient in regard to beliefs, cognitive abilities, and social background?

Patient-Centered Standard

What perhaps is needed is a **Patient–Centered Standard** that relies on the unique nature and abilities of the individual patient to determine the amount of disclosure needed to satisfy the requirements of informed consent. This more subjective standard would allow a greater differentiation based on patient-reference. A patient who values a pain-free life is very different from one who values an extended life regardless of pain, or as in the case of the would-be great author, a person who values a life with full faculties above all other considerations is possibly quite different from some hypothetical reasonable patient.

In practice, the courts have not provided clear direction, inasmuch as they can be seen at various times to be forceful proponents for both autonomy and paternalism. In several landmark cases, an absolute need for individual self-determination, with the requirements of informed consent, has been outlined; while in others, the doors have been opened for therapeutic privilege and professional determination. *Therapeutic privilege* is the legal exception to the rule of informed consent, which allows the care giver to proceed with care without consent in cases of emergency, incompetence, and where, due to depression or instability, the patient could be harmed by the information. The latter case is a rather controversial form of therapeutic privilege, as the decision to withhold information based on "sound medical judgment" opens the door for professional determinism at the expense of patient autonomy.

This shifting in position can be highlighted in the difference between the early cases of *Pratt v. Davis* (1905),[9] and *Schloendorff v. The Society of New York Hospital* (1914),[10] as well as later cases such as *Canterbury v. Spence* (1972).[8] In the two early cases the courts outlined a rigid respect for personal autonomy: "Under a free government at least, the free citizen's first and greatest right which underlies all the others—the right to the inviolability of his person, in other words, his right to himself . . . ."[10] This right to self was supreme even if the physician was attempting to do good. Doing good was not enough if the good was performed without the consent of the patient. In the Schloendorff case, a woman had refused surgery but had allowed the physician to examine her under ether. During the examination, the surgeon had found fibroid tumors that needed to be removed, and proceeded to remove them, feeling that the care was medically expedient. In his review, Justice Cardozo wrote:

> Every human being of adult years and sound mind has a right to determine what shall be done with his own body; and a surgeon who performs an operation without his patient's consent, commits an assault for which he is liable in damages."[10]

In later cases, the courts have moved away from a rigid defense of autonomy and allowed for a level of benevolent deception. The *Canterbury v. Spence* case involved a 19-year-old male who underwent a laminectomy for severe back pain. After the surgery, he attempted without assistance, to get up to urinate. In his attempt, he fell and suffered a setback that lead to paralysis from the waist down. Although he had been warned about moving without assistance, he sued on the basis of negligent failure to warn him of the risk of paralysis.

Although the court was deeply sympathetic to the young man, it held that the physician had not been negligent in failing to explain the risk of paralysis, and that if, in his or her medical judgment, the patient was better served by the deception, under the empowerment of therapeutic privilege the physician could limit the amount of disclosure.

> It is recognized that patients occasionally become so ill or distraught on disclosure as to foreclose a rational decision, or complicate or hinder the treatment, or perhaps even pose psychological damage to the patient. . . . The critical inquiry is whether the physician responded to a sound medical judgment that communication of the risk information would present a threat to the patient's well being.[8]

The courts have not provided a consistent presentation of what is required in regard to informed consent, at times seeming to shift from full disclosure to the allowance of paternalism. Critics such as Jay Katz [11] have likened informed consent to a fairy tale. He argues that, although the doctrine is enchantingly appealing in its simplicity, it does not live up to its promise of delivering decisional authority to the patients. The reality of current medical practice does not fulfill the promise, and is often perfunctorily performed, not so much to convey information and open dialog between physicians and patients as to comply with the legal letter of the law. Katz argues that "once kissed by the doctrine, frog-patients" do not become "autonomous princes."

COMPETENCY DETERMINATION

What, then, is the basis of the medical judgment that overcomes and limits patient autonomy? As a general rule, the practitioner must respect and abide by the decisions of an autonomous patient. This general rule, however, cannot apply when the patient's decision is based on incomplete information, lack of understanding, or external controlling influences that preclude independent judgment. Figure 4–2 outlines the moral and relevant factors that often influence physicians' decisions in regard to honoring the wishes of the critically ill. [12]

If we examine the case of a young man injured shortly after returning home from war, we can see the effects of the six factors (Fig. 4–2) in play. In this case, the

1. The patient's ability to make choices about care. Does the patient have sufficient information and intellectual capacity to make rational choices?
2. The patient's consistency with his own values. Are the choices made by the patient authentic in the sense of being consistent with his own values? Are the choices sufficiently independent of and not controlled by others?
3. Age. It would seem that a more mature patient's refusal in life-threatening circumstances can often be more easily respected than the refusal of a much younger person.
4. Nature of the illness. Whether the illness can be diagnosed and what the prognosis is can be significant, especially if complete recovery is possible with appropriate treatment.
5. The attitudes and values of the physician responsible for the decision. The physician's moral and religious background, as well as attitudes toward life and death have a role to play in the physician's choice.
6. The clinical setting. When authority is diffused among a health care team, decisions must be reached in a different way from those used in such private settings as the physician's office or the patient's home.

FIGURE 4–2 Common factors used in decisions regarding patient competence

individual, a hometown war hero, while waiting for an opportunity to begin a career as a commercial pilot, was involved in an oil field/natural gas accident that left him severely burned, disfigured, blind, and without the use of his hands. Although the young man was badly injured, it became apparent that he would survive and that his claim against the petrochemical company was such that he would never, under reasonable circumstances, be in financial need.

Early in his care, it became apparent to the young man that he was facing an extended period of rehabilitation and treatment for his burns. At this time, he came to the decision that he did not want to continue the painful treatment or to live the life of a blind disfigured person.

At this early stage of care, it could be concluded that the pain and medications had precluded the young man from making a rational **authentic decision** in regard to stopping treatment. If allowed, his decision to stop treatment would have meant an early death due to infection. Using Factor 1 (the patient's ability to make choices about care), the medical staff could decide that the pain and medications could be limiting his ability to make a rational choice and, therefore, continue the care despite his protestations. Using the patient's blindness and physical handicap as a rationale, the physicians authorized his mother to sign the consent forms for the continuation of his care.

As time went on and the young man continued to protest medical care, the physicians had him undergo psychiatric evaluation to determine his competence. The results of this evaluation were that, indeed, the patient was competent and that the decision was authentic: He did not wish the care based on his evaluation that the pain of the treatment was greater than the value of his future life. The patient did not value a life that left him disfigured, blind, and without the use of his hands.

At this time if the physicians had attended to Factors 2 (authentic decision), 3 (age), or 4 (prognosis of condition), they might have allowed for the patient's self-determination, as the decision appeared authentic, his maturity was not in question, and the nature of the prognosis was such that he would not be returned to a state of health that he valued. However, the actual decision, which was to continue the treatment, seems more based on Factors 5 (attitude and values of the physician) and 6 (clinical setting). The decision rested not upon the desires of the patient or his **competency**, but rather upon the physician's personal values, and those of his mother and lawyer, as well as the institutional decision-making system. The treatment was continued, although the patient was somewhat mollified by the idea that, if he would put up with the treatment, he could later make his own decisions in regard to ending his life without constraint.

This case points out that the factors outlined in Figure 4–2 do indeed represent considerations used by physicians for decision making, but provide no clear mechanism for the decisions themselves. If we intend to honor the autonomy of our patients, then only Factors 1 (ability to make decision), 2 (authentic decision), and 3 (age) need be considered. What seems to be needed is a systematic method by which the focus of the decision-making process is patient based. The real questions that need to be addressed are: Is the patient in a position to make an authentic decision, and should we allow the patient to make this decision under these circumstances?

With certain categories of individuals, such as children, the mentally incompetent, and those coerced by pain or trauma to the point of incapacity for rational reasoning, the decision to limit personal autonomy is rather an easy one, and often made.

In general, a competent adult has the absolute right to refuse medical treatment even if the refusal is life threatening. At question is patient autonomy, which is positively confirmed by being able to answer yes to two questions: (1) Does the patient understand the nature of the illness, and the consequences of the various options that may be chosen? and (2) Is the decision based on rational reasoning? The decision itself need not be rational but the reasoning process should be. Given First Amendment protections for religious belief, the second question in regard to the need for rational processes needs to be modified to include the protection of decisions based on faith, i.e., "a belief held to be true, in regard to things unseen." A corollary question needs to be added in these cases: (3) Is this seemingly irrational thinking based on a religious belief acceptable and entitled to First Amendment protections? In order to be protected, a belief must be held by a sufficient number of people, for an extended time period, or be sufficiently like other beliefs that are held by other groups that are considered orthodox.

In regard to the Jehovah's Witness faith, the courts have provided a rather inconsistent picture in regard to honoring the decision not to accept transfusions. Orthodox Jehovah's Witnesses believe that in the Old and New Testament Scriptures, the Lord declares that His followers should not partake of blood:[13]

> The life of every creature is in its blood. That is why I have said to the Israelites, "you must not eat the blood of any creature . . . anyone who eats it must be cut off" (Lev. 17: 13–14).
>   . . . abstain from food pulluted by idols, from sexually immorality, from the meat of strangled animals and from blood (Acts 15:20).

To Witnesses, the acceptance of a transfusion places them in a situation where they may indeed prolong their life here on earth, but places them in jeopardy of being eternally *cut off* from their God.

The decision to honor decisions of this nature is not based on whether an individual's faith is rational to the health care provider, but rather on whether the decision is being make by an autonomous adult. In a 1965 Chicago case in which a woman repeatedly told her physician that she understood the consequences of her actions, but as an act of faith could not take a transfusion, the courts held:

> Even though we may consider the appellant's beliefs unwise, foolish or ridiculous, in the absence of an overriding danger to society we may not permit interference . . . in the waning hours of her life for the sole purpose of compelling her to accept medical treatment forbidden by her religious principles and previously refused by her with full knowledge of the probable consequence.[14]

The decision by an autonomous Jehovah's Witness patient not to accept a lifesaving blood transfusion could be honored. We would do so on the basis that they understand the nature of the condition and the consequences of their options, thereby satisfying Question 1. They would need to rely on First Amendment protection of their rights, as the decision is not a matter of reason but faith, using the corollary to Question 2. It is interesting that if the patient appealed not to a protected orthodoxy but rather to someone like the "First Poo Baa of Mu," who dwells under Mt. Shasta, we would consider the decision delusionary and would limit the autonomy in order to protect the patient.

Even in protected beliefs however, patients must satisfy the requirements of Question 1, in that they must understand the nature of their condition and the consequences of the various options. An individual who states that by failing to be treated, he knows that he will be healed and not face death, has not met the requirements of knowing and accepting the potential consequences of his actions. This is a much different case than that of another person who tells you that, yes indeed, she understands that she may die as a result of her decision to refuse treatment, but feels that the need to follow the dictates of her particular faith is such that she will place her fate in the hands of God.

The autonomy of members of the Jehovah's Witness faith or other orthodox religion that restricts medical care does not extend to the refusing of medical care for their children. The courts have held that parents no longer exercise the power of life and death over a child.

> Parents may be free to become martyrs themselves. But it does not follow that they are free . . . to make martyrs of their children before the children reach the age of full and legal discretion when they can make that choice for themselves.[15]

In these cases the courts will usually appoint a guardian **ad litem** for the specific and limited purpose of making treatment decisions on behalf of the child. The child is usually not removed from the home or control of the parents except for the limited area of medical decision making.

In nursing homes across the United States, there are estimated to be 80,000 patients with some level of dementia. Most of them, following our guidelines, would be determined incompetent to make decisions in regard to their medical care. In the acute hospital setting, about 50 percent of the decisions not to resuscitate if the patient begins to fail involve incompetent patients. The question of competency determination, and who makes the decisions when incompetence is determined, is a problem that will continue to bedevil modern medical care until systems are developed to handle these cases. The outlines of such a system will be handled in later chapters.

SUMMARY

The providing of health care is a shared practice, in which the expert and the consumer both work to be sure that what is delivered is satisfactory to each. As the expert, the practitioner knows what is needed in a pure medical sense, but does not know how the value preferences of the patient will affect what part of the care will be accepted.

Since there is general agreement that, through the exercise of personal autonomy, the patient has the right to decide the nature of care, it is vital that the practitioner make sure that the decision is based on appropriate information. Informed consent is required for all invasive or risky procedures that have potential for harm. The physician must disclose pertinent details about the nature and purpose of the procedure, its risks and benefits, and any reasonable alternatives to the recommended treatment.

There have been several standards for this disclosure of information, but today most practitioners recognize the reasonable patient standard, which requires that the information be explained in such a manner that a hypothetical reasonable person could understand and make decisions. Because all of us are unique in what we value, it may be time to develop a more subjective standard than that of a "reasonable person".

While there is general agreement that the autonomous adult has the right to decide these issues, there are times when the autonomy of the patient is limited by pain, trauma, age, and mental competency. Competency is usually established in the ability to answer two questions in the affirmative: First, does the patient understand the nature of the condition and the various options available; and, second, is the decision-making process rational? The second question is somewhat modified when the decision is based on a protected religious faith, rather than reason.

Paternalism in its best sense is based on the principle of beneficence and a desire to do well for the patient. In modern health care, this desire to do good is not a justification for overcoming a competent patient's personal autonomy.

CLARIFICATION EXERCISES

A. Often decisions in regard to accepting or rejecting health care are dependent not on medical expertise but rather on the value preferences of the patient. The following list of values in regard to health might cause very different decisions in regard to care. Rank-order the list in terms of importance to you personally.

    1. "I want to live as long as possible."_____

    2. "I wouldn't want to live if I were on a ventilator."_____

    3. "If I can't live an active life, I don't want to live at all."_____

    4. "I don't care what you do, or what condition I'm in, as long as I don't suffer from any pain."_____

    5. "I would rather die than live a life that doesn't allow me to be me."_____

    In regard to the case of the author with a terminal disease, which of the above values best express his decision?_____

B. The following cases are examples of the struggle between patient autonomy and the directive to do good and avoid harm. State what you think should be done in each case.

    1. A young woman in the early stages of pregnancy has a mild but not disfiguring case of acne. She has recently read that a new medication will cure the condition and requests a prescription. By consulting the *Physicians' Desk Reference* outlining the effects of the medication, the physician finds that the drug has the potential for teratogenic effect and might harm the fetus. He informs the patient of the problem; however, the woman wants to take the chance and demands a prescription for the new medication.

2. Mr. Green, a middle-aged man with a family history of heart disease, including the untimely death of his father and uncles, begins to become short winded upon moderate exercise. He is very frightened and has a morbid fear that perhaps he is beginning to have the same problems as his relatives.

   After Mr. Green has been examined by his physician, he tells her that he does not want to know the truth if the results are bad. The examination results show that, indeed, he has serious problems and will likely suffer a major heart attack unless he agrees to immediate surgery and a change in lifestyle.

3. Mrs. Smith, a young woman 32 years of age with two children, is a member of the Jehovah's Witness faith. After a serious automobile accident, she has internal bleeding that appears to be life threatening. The physician wishes to transfuse the patient in order to stabilize her so that exploratory surgery can be done and the bleeding halted. The patient refuses the treatment, based on her belief that it would be against the will of God.

   Following are two ways in which the patient's decision might be framed. One would be acceptable in regard to competency determination and the other would not. Decide which could be honored as an authentic autonomous decision, and which could not. Defend your decision.

   (a) "I refuse this blood, as it is against my religion. I feel that the taking of blood is against the will of God. I understand the consequences of this decision and am willing to place my fate in the hands of my God, who will bless me and be merciful."

   (b) "I refuse this blood, as it is against my religion. I feel that the taking of blood is against the will of God. I know that if I am faithful to His will, He will bless me with a long life and the opportunity to raise my children."

   We can see similar reasoning in the decision in the *Department of Human Services v. Northern* case (563 SW2d 197, 1978), where a lucid, intelligent, 72-year-old female patient expressed the desire to both live and keep her gangrenous foot. In that keeping the gangrenous foot was not compatable with living, the court held that she was delusional and ordered protective services on her behalf.

4. Mr. Jones is an active, elderly man (80 years of age) in a nursing home who has no close relatives except a young nephew. During a walk one day, he receives a puncture wound to the leg that becomes infected and gangrenous. As a result of his illness, Mr. Jones has a high fever and becomes unresponsive to questions. The physician decides that the only way to save his life is to remove his leg. The nephew tells the physician that he does not think his uncle would want to live if his leg were amputated. The patient has left no advanced directives in regard to what he would wish in such a case.
   • Before you come to a conclusion in this case you will need to investigate all the facts—usually of the who, what, why, when, and how variety. In making your decision in regard to Mr. Jones, list the questions you would like answered and the individuals you would like to discuss the case with (for example, the head nurse of the unit).
   • When you question Mr. Jones's lawyer you are told that the nephew is his only heir and that he is very wealthy. Does this change your decision?
   • Once all the facts of the case have been examined and the motivations of the individuals explored, the next phase of decision making is to generate all the solutions of initial credibility. In regard to Mr. Jones, list these. Now estimate how each of your solutions would affect each of the following individuals: Mr. Jones, the nephew, the physician.
   • State your decision and evaluate it in regard to the basic principles involved. Does it promote them or sacrifice them?

C. You are a radiographer doing an ultrasound examination on a pregnant patient, and the woman wants the test to determine the week of gestation so that she can determine whether she can legally request an abortion. If your personal view is that of "pro-life" would you need to perform the test? What place does your professional autonomy play?

D. What information needed to be explained to the 19-year-old in the *Canterbury v. Spence* case to assure that the requirements of informed consent had been complied with?

E. In the legal case *Stepp v. Review Board of the Indiana Employment Security Division* (521 NE 2d 350, (Ind Ct App. 1988), a laboratory technician was found to have been properly dismissed from her job for refusing to perform chemical examinations on vials with AIDS warnings attached. If professionals have the right to professional autonomy, shouldn't the technician have been allowed to refuse to provide the service? Whatever your opinion, defend your position.

F. In a recent article, Ezekial and Linda Emanuel have proposed four models of the physician-patient relationship.[16] Compare and contrast these four models with those offered by Robert Veatch and described earlier in this chapter.

Paternalistic Model: In this model, the interaction is designed to assure that the patient makes the decision that best promotes his or her health and well-being. The health care provider presents selected information in such a way as to encourage consent to the intervention that is most medically appropriate. The health care provider is functioning in the role of a guardian.

Informative Model: The health care provider in this case supplies the patient with all relevant information and allows the patient to select the intervention he or she wishes. The concept is rooted in the idea that the patient knows his or her own value system and needs only receive the facts in order to make an appropriate, patient-centered decision. The health care provider in these interactions is functioning in the role of technical specialist.

Interpretive Model: The interaction in this model is designed to elucidate the patient's values and what he or she really wants, then to help that patient select the interventions compatible with those values. The health care provider is functioning in the role of a counselor or advisor.

Deliberative Model: Under this model, the health care provider seeks to help the patient determine and chose the best health-care related values that can be realized in the particular clinical situation. The health care provider helps the patient in value clarification as well as in understanding the aspects of the various potential interventions. The provider discusses not only what the patient could do but also what the patient should do in the situation. The health care provider serves as a teacher and friend in this model.

Which of these models do you feel best serves the interest of your patient group and is most ethical in regard to respecting both patient autonomy and our duty to the principle of beneficence? Explain your decision.

REFERENCES AND SUGGESTED READING

1. American Medical Association, *Code of Ethics* (1848).
2. *A Patient's Bill of Rights,* statement issued by the American Hospital Association and affirmed by the AHA House of Delegates on February 6, 1973.
3. John Stuart Mill, *On Liberty,* ed. Gertrude Himmelfarb (New York: Penguin Books, 1974), pp. 68–69.
4. Pedro lain Entralgo, "What does the word 'Good' mean in 'Good Patient,'" in *Changing Values in Medicine,* ed. E. Cassel, and M. Siegler (New York: University Publications of America, 1979) pp. 127–145.
5. Robert Veatch, *A Theory of Medical Ethics* (New York: Masik Books Inc., 1981).
6. Gary Anderson and Valerie Anderson, *Health Care Ethics* (Rockville, MD: An Aspen Publication, 1987), pp. 199–200.

7. *Natanson v. Kline*, 186 Kansas 393 P2d 1093 (1960).

8. *Canterbury v. Spence*, 464 F2d 772, at 785–787 (DC Cir 1972).

9. *Pratt v. Davis*, 118 Illinois App 161 (1905).

10. *Schloendorff v. New York Hospital*, 211 New York 125, 105 NE, 92, 93 (1914).

11. Jay Katz, "Informed Consent—A Fairy Tale? in T. Beauchamp and L. Walters, *Contemporary Issues in Bioethics* (Belmont, CA: Wadsworth Press, 1982) pp. 191–197.

12. Mark Siegler, "Critical Illness: The Limits of Autonomy," *The Hastings Center Report* 7 (October 1977), 12–15.

13. Leviticus 17: 13–14, Acts 15:20, Old and New Testament, *King James Version of Bible*.

14. In re *Estate of Brooks*, 32 Illinois 2d 361, 205 NE (1965).

15. *Prince v. Mass.* 321 US 158, 166 (1944).

16. E. Emanuel and L. Emanuel, "Four Models of the Physician-Patient Relationship," *Journal of the American Medical Association* 267, no. 16: 2221–2226.

———— CHAPTER 5 ————

CONFIDENTIALITY AND THE MANAGEMENT OF HEALTH CARE INFORMATION

Instructional Goal

The major instructional goal for this chapter is to gain an understanding of the current problems associated with the principle of confidentiality as it is applied in modern health care.

Instructional Objectives

At the end of this chapter the reader should understand and be able to:

1. Write a defense for the principle of confidentiality within health care from a utilitarian, duty-oriented, and virtue ethics point of view.
2. Explain the rationale for "the Harm principle" as it relates to the Tarasoff case.
3. List the two basic principles in conflict in the Tarasoff case.
4. Give five instances in which the practitioner would have a legal requirement to report confidential matters that relate to health care.
5. Explain how vulnerability guides the decision-making process when confidentiality is overridden by the duty to warn.
6. List five groups, not involved in direct patient care, who have a legitimate interest in the medical record.

7. List six safeguards that should be considered in regard to allowing access to confidential patient information.

8. Explain why confidentiality is considered a principle with qualifications.

Glossary

Harm Principle: When the practitioner can foresee a danger to an individual who is outside the patient/provider relationship, potentially caused by the patient, the harm principle provides the rationale for breaching confidentiality to warn the vulnerable individual.

Institutional Review Boards: Review boards that examine the protocol design for research to assure that the research conforms to appropriate standards.

Right to Privacy: The right to be left alone; the right of a person to be free from unwarranted publicity.

Third-Party Payers: Agencies such as insurance companies or governmental programs that are called upon to pay for health care services.

Utilization Review: A review of the appropriateness of care and the various types of patient care provided within an institution. It is usually designed to assure appropriate and cost-effective care.

CONFIDENTIALITY: A PRINCIPLE WITH QUALIFICATIONS

The patient has a right to every consideration of privacy concerning his own medical care program. Case discussion, consultation, examination, and treatment are confidential and should be conducted discreetly. Those not directly involved in his care must have the permission of the patient to be present. The patient has the right to expect that all communications and records pertaining to his care should be treated as confidential.

A Patient's Bill of Rights

A patient's basic right to expect the information he gives a health care practitioner to be held in confidence can be arrived at and defended using any of the three systematic approaches to ethical decision making outlined in Chapter 2. Whether the reasoning is from a utilitarian, duty-oriented, or virtue ethics standpoint, confidentiality seems to be a settled issue.

From a utilitarian point of view, the long-term consequences of making public any personal information gained as a result of the practitioner/patient relationship would have a chilling effect upon the truth-telling in that relationship. Since health care practice is normally conducted under a tacit agreement of confidentiality, practitioners who breach this trust are in violation of an agreed-upon expectation. This is especially critical in psychotherapy, where the patient is encouraged to take the risks involved in personal disclosure. If the patient has lost confidence in the process, and fails to discuss personal issues with the practitioner, the amount of care that can be provided will be severely limited.

From a duty-oriented perspective, personal privacy is a basic right, with its foundations firmly based not only in long-standing codes of professional practice but also in common law. The unwarranted disclosure of a patient's private affairs, the unauthorized use of a person's photograph, or exploitation of a person's name have traditionally been considered acts that might give rise to legal action, on the grounds of invasion of an individual's right to privacy. The legal standard for judging a breach of confidence is clear: You may be found liable for any unauthorized breach of confidentiality that "offends the sensibilities of an ordinary person."[1] The medical duty to protect the confidentiality of patients could be argued on the basis of our general rights as citizens to be free from invasion of privacy. The individual in our society has the autonomous right to the control of personal information and the protection of personal privacy. In some sense, privacy can be viewed as a person's right, while confidentiality is the professional's duty.

From the vantage point of virtue ethics, the practice of patient confidentiality has been a mainstay of health care practice and forms one of the virtues that one would expect from the "good practitioner." Figure 5–1 outlines the requirements of this principle as found in the Hippocratic Oath.

Confidentiality is a critical principle, and, regardless of the specialty, the "good practitioner" cannot be viewed as cavalier in regard to protecting patients' confidences and privacy. While it is obvious that confidential information must be shared among practitioners in order to provide the best care for the patient or to extend the body of knowledge within health care, it is equally obvious that this does not take the form of conversations in elevators, in cafeterias, or with friends at a party.

The real question, then, is not whether confidentiality is a good—regardless of what reasoning you use—but whether it is a moral absolute, or might be overridden by other considerations. In the classic Tarasoff case, a young man by the name of Prosenjit Poddar confided to his clinical psychologist that he intended to kill a young woman he readily identified as Tatiana. The psychologist, understanding that his patient presented a real danger to the young woman, decided that Prosenjit should

---

"What I may see or hear in the course of treatment or even outside of treatment in regard to the life of men, which on no account must be noised abroad, I will keep to myself holding such things shameful to be spoken about."

Hippocratic Oath

FIGURE 5–1 Confidentiality

be committed for 72 hours to allow further evaluation, and he notified security to assist in securing the patient's confinement.

The patient, however, convinced the security officers that he was rational, and he was released following his promise to stay away from the young woman. The health care providers rescinded the orders to place Prosenjit in confinement for evaluation, and no efforts were made to warn Tatiana or her family of potential danger. Within weeks of these events, Prosenjit murdered the young woman.[2]

The health care practitioners later defended their decision to maintain patient confidentiality on the basis that they had a duty only to their patient, and in the absence of duty they were not required to protect the life and safety of others. To whom did the caregivers owe duty, to their real patient or to the potential victim? They had chosen to serve the one and ignore the other. Arguments used in their defense were that effective treatment required the patient's full disclosure of his innermost thoughts, and that, without the promise of confidentiality, patients needing treatment would fail to seek care.

In it's decision, the court recognized the difficulty that a practitioner might have in attempting to predict whether statements made by a patient would be actually carried out. However, the court ruled that the specialist would be held to the standard of reasonable practice, and where that standard indicated a foreseeable danger to another, a duty to warn was created. The protective privilege of confidentiality is limited where the health and safety of others is involved. This breaching of the trust of confidentiality is recognized and allowed by the Principles of Medical Ethics of the American Medical Association, which states that.

> A physician may not reveal the confidences entrusted to him in the course of medical attendance . . . , unless he is required to do so by law or unless it becomes necessary in order to protect the welfare of the individual or of the community.

The balance between protecting the confidentiality of the patients we serve and yet safeguarding the community has found its way into many specialties' codes of ethics. This balance can be seen in the guideline for confidentiality for the Colorado Society of Clinical Specialists in Psychiatric Nursing, as adopted in 1987:

Confidentiality

1. Keep all client records secure.
2. Consider carefully the content to be entered into the record.
3. Release information only with written consent and full discussion of the information to be shared, except when release is required by law.
4. Use professional judgment deliberately regarding confidentiality when the client is a danger to self or others.
5. Use professional judgment deliberately when deciding how to maintain the confidentiality of a minor. The rights of the parent/guardian must also be considered.
6. Disguise clinical material when used professionally for teaching and writing.[3]

In her book *Secrets: On the Ethics of Concealment and Revelation,* Sissela Bok cites several instances where confidentiality is overridden by more compelling obligations.[4] Many of these have found their way into legal statutes, and practitioners are generally required to report cases involving child abuse, contagious diseases, sexually transmitted diseases, wounds caused by guns or knives, and other cases where identifiable third parties would be placed at risk by failure to disclose the information. Bok feels that the personal protective privilege of confidentiality is limited by the **harm principle.** This principle requires that health care providers refrain from acts or omissions that would foreseeably result in harm to others, especially in those cases where the individuals are particularly vulnerable to the risk.

An example of the how the harm principle is modified by vulnerability might be provided by the case of a married man who tests HIV positive. In that the risk to the community at large is rather minimal, whereas the risk to the man in regard to discrimination, deprivation of rights, and occupational and social harm are great, the practitioner would have an obligation to be very discrete in regard to confidentiality, and to do little more than that which is legally required in reporting the test results. However, in the case of the wife, who is far more vulnerable than the community at large, the practitioner must either be assured that the situation is modified in order to lessen the woman's vulnerability or disclose the information to the woman. It would seem, then, that the practitioner's observance of the principle of confidentiality must always be balanced by the need to protect others from foreseeable harm especially if the other individual is particularly vulnerable to that harm.[4]

MODERN HEALTH CARE AND CONFIDENTIALITY

In the early 1900s, maintaining confidentiality was a much easier task, as 85 percent of the direct medical care services were delivered by physicians. Access to medical records and the obligation to maintain confidentiality in regard to them was limited to the physician and a very small direct staff. Today over 80 percent of direct patient care is provided by allied health and nursing professionals. In the hospital, only about a third of the patient record is maintained by physicians, with the rest being recorded by other members of the health care team.[5]

The patient record is not only accessible to the attending physicians but also is readily available to a host of technical and administrative staff who generate and handle patient data. Following the complaint of one patient in regard to confidentiality, a survey revealed that at least 75 individuals had legitimate access to the patient's record by virtue of the fact that they were involved in providing either direct care or support services.

Moreover, the problem of access to patient information has been exacerbated by the growing use of computerized information systems. The large scale on which information can be stored and the ease of access to these data have made distribution of the information outside the arena of the patient/health care practitioner interface a daily routine, as patient data are used for administration, payment, **utilization review,** teaching, and research. In addition to the health care providers, patient files may be available to the following: insurance companies, (because they pay the bills), public health agencies (to assist in monitoring and investigating disease outbreak patterns), employers (to assess job-related injuries) federal, state, and local government (to develop health care plans and to allocate resources), attorneys and law enforcement agencies (as evidence to settle civil and/or criminal matters), media (to report health hazards and to help report medical research development), and accreditation, licensing, and certification agencies (to assess compliance with various criteria and standards.[6]

The concerns of these **third-party payers** with access to medical information may or may not coincide with the patient's best interests, inasmuch as confidentiality and privacy are not necessarily a high priority for groups such as governmental regulators, third-party payers, insurers, or utilization reviewers. Given the tasks they perform, they may favor safety, truth, and knowledge far more than they value the personal privacy of a single patient. The computerized accumulation, analysis, and storage of unlimited quantities of medical information have overwhelmed the medical record professionals who are entrusted with protecting patient privacy and confidentiality. Mark Siegler, Director of the Center for Clinical Medical Ethics at the University of Chicago, argues that in hospital medicine, the existence of third-party interests and the development of the team medicine has made confidentiality a "decrepit concept."[7]

LEGAL PERSPECTIVE TO MEDICAL RECORD ACCESS

Many state statutes and a few federal regulations require the reporting of certain types of information, from the medical record, to appropriate agencies with or without the patient's authorization. Often these reporting requirements deal with issues vital to community health and welfare, such as child abuse, poison and industrial accidents, communicable diseases, misadministration of radioactive materials, blood transfusion reactions, injuries with guns or knives, and narcotic use. The child abuse statutes in most states require that hospitals and practitioners report incidents of suspected abuse. In these cases, the practitioners are protected from liability if they are making the report in good faith even if the reported abuse proves to be false. Failure to make a report in regard to child abuse by those required to do so can leave them legally liable for any additional injuries the child may suffer upon return to the hostile home environment. An Illinois statute is illustrative:

> Any physician, hospital administrator and personnel engaged in examination, care and treatments of persons, . . . having reasonable cause to believe a child known to them in their professional or official capacity may be an abused child or a neglected child shall immediately report or cause a report to be made . . . The privileged quality of communication between any professional person required to report and his patient or client shall not apply to situations involving abused or neglected children and shall not constitute grounds for failure to report as required by this Act.[8]

Some states maintain a registry of the names and addresses of all patients who obtain drugs that are subject to abuse. These reporting regulations have been upheld as a reasonable exercise of an individual state's broad police powers. In the absence of a legal regulation to provide patient information, a police agency has no authority to examine a medical record without the patient's authorization.

LEGITIMATE INTEREST

The medical record goes far beyond just medical information and contains personal data of a financial and social nature. In general, it is the property of the hospital or clinic, but the patient has a legal interest and right to the information. It is generally considered that the record is confidential and that access to it should be limited to the patient, authorized representatives of the patient, the attending physician, and hospital staff members who have a legitimate interest. The exact specification of who has a legitimate interest is a great concern to health care practitioners, but some general guidelines are accepted where the need is for patient care, professional education, administrative functions, auditing functions, research, public health reporting, and criminal law requirements. In regard to patient care, any information may be shared among health care providers who are responsible for the patient within the treating facility. Modern medicine is a team practice, and adequate exchange of information is necessary for patient care.

The need for professional education usually permits information in regard to in-house patients to be exchanged for these purposes. This generally includes medicine, nursing, allied health, psychology, social services, or any other professional group involved in the patient care. If the information is to be disseminated outside the treating facility (as in a patient case study), this may not be done without prior patient consent or unless the information is in a form that precludes all possible patient identification.

Limited amounts of information as needed for the administrative functions of appointments, admissions, discharges, billing, compiling census data, and the like are necessarily shared among clerical and administrative staff.

Duly appointed quality-of-care auditors, governmental third-party payers, and professional review organizations have a legitimate access to the patient record. The Peer Review Organization (PRO) program, which replaced the Professional Standards Review Organization (PSRO) program in 1982, requires that the PROs disclose review information according to guidelines set forth by the Department of Health and Human Services. This information is reported to: (1) state and federal fraud and abuse agencies; (2) agencies responsible for identification of public health problems; and (3) state licenser and certification agencies.

Data in regard to the conducting of research can generally be shared with all the researchers involved, provided that the patient is not identified directly or indirectly in the process, or subsequently in any other report or presentation. Hospitals that permit their staff to engage in research generally have research committees set up to screen the protocols. These **institutional review boards** (IRBs) attempt to balance the potential risk to the patient against the potential benefits of the research. In the absence of more stringent standards, the research committees should require the following as minimum standards:[9]

1. The research results should be presented in such a fashion as to protect the anonymity of the patients.

2. Only those involved in the study will have access to the raw data.

3. Safeguards to protect the patient's privacy will be part of the research protocol.

4. The same level of obligation to maintain patient confidentiality in the practice of health care is expected in the conduct of medical research.

Health care providers often record far more than is needed for documentation or to convey the necessary information required for patient care. It generally is not necessary for confidences to be recorded in explicit detail. A note in the record that a young patient "has a close relationship" with her boyfriend, would generally be adequate to jog the practitioner's memory in regard to the need for counseling of a sexually active teenager. The less confidential information written explicitly into the record, the fewer opportunities for harmful disclosures involving patient privacy. Only material necessary for documentation and therapeutic care should be recorded, for example, in the case of a stab wound, the practitioner would not necessarily confide to the record other privileged information in regard to the attack on prior crimes or involvement in gang warfare.

The Patient's Bill of Rights, provided by the American Hospital Association, outlines patients' right to inspect their own charts and to receive complete information concerning their treatment in the hospital. In some states, the rules governing access to the medical records of mental health patients differ from those of the general patient population. In the past, these patients were not given access to their records—a practice based on the assumption that access would be injurious to their health. However, recent court cases have tended toward allowing this patient group to have greater access to their records, and in some states mental health patients have the same right to inspect their records as do other patient populations.

It is essential that hospitals establish effective procedures to protect the content of medical records, not only from the standpoint of patient confidentiality, but also against the possibility of intentional falsification or alteration of the record. Unfortunately, records have been doctored by patients and practitioners alike who wished to improve their chances in pending legal actions. To protect the security of their medical records the following minimal guidelines are suggested:

• Competent medical records or risk-management personnel should review a record before it is examined by the patient or the patient's representative.

• An original medical record should not be permitted to be taken from the hospital's premises except pursuant to legal process or a defined hospital procedure, such as allowing an accompanied patient to transport records to another facility for testing purposes.

• Neither the patient nor the patient's authorized representative is to be allowed to examine the medical records alone.[9]

SUMMARY

Personal privacy appears to be under siege in all aspects of our lives. The use of computers has greatly increased this concern, as it is common knowledge that all of us have dossiers in several major data banks. These governmental and commercial data sources provide information to others in regard to credit ratings, marital status, and even hobbies and interests. It seems at times that one need only provide a small donation to a favorite charity (perhaps to save the woodlands) before being inundated by an avalanche of offers for the type of person who might want to save woodlands, or at least look woodsy.

The general patient population still places a great deal of faith in the manner in which health care providers maintain the principle of confidentiality. Confidentiality seems to serve two basic purposes. First, the principle acknowledges a respect for the individual's **right to privacy** as guaranteed by our legal system and enshrined in our cultural values. Second, and perhaps more important to the health of the patient, the promise of confidentiality provides a bond between the practitioner and patient that allows for a full and honest disclosure of information. In those rare cases where disclosure is necessary to protect a community interest, confidentiality must be balanced by a duty to warn, especially with vulnerable third parties.

Although the establishment of hospital team medicine and bureaucratic interventions has eroded the principle of confidentiality, it is imperative that, to the fullest possible extent, health care providers take meticulous care to guarantee that patients' medical and personal information be kept confidential. To the degree that health care providers must breach confidentiality to third parties, it would seem that the patient should be notified of the nature and ramifications of these disclosures. If patients understand what will happen to the information, they then would be in a better position to decide which of their personal matters they would chose to relate and what they would prefer to keep private.

Policies must be designed to balance the right to legitimate personal privacy while not offsetting the institutional need to make necessary information quickly and easily available to those who have a legitimate claim to it. It would seem that, at a minimum, these privacy safeguards should: (1) define circumstances under which medical information is disclosed to other parties; (2) provide procedures by which patients may gain access to their records; (3) allow access to records to others only on a "need to know" basis; (4) ensure anonymity in aggregating data for research or statistical purposes; (5) carefully balance society's long-term goals and the legitimate need of organizations to have access to medical records with the patient's short-term desire for and right to privacy; and (6) inform the patient of what is meant by confidentiality in the context of current practice.

These safeguards would be in the spirit of informed consent and would offer some protection against misuse and abuse of patient information. In addition, if patients have access to their records, they can ensure that the information contained therein is accurate, complete, and relevant to their care. Patient advocacy is a significant responsibility of health care practitioners, and the restoration of some semblance of institutional responsibility in the area of confidentiality is necessary if our patients are to continue to believe in the process.

CLARIFICATION EXERCISES

A. Unauthorized vs. authorized disclosure: In this exercise state whether you think the disclosure of information was appropriate or inappropriate and defend your position.

1. A young woman who states she has just been raped comes into the emergency room requesting a pelvic examination and a morning-after pill but insists that the staff not call the police. The staff reports the incident.

2. A young father brings his child into the emergency room for treatment of an arm injury. The family has brought the child in several times, of late, for similar injuries with the excuse that she is somewhat clumsy and is having difficulty learning to ride her bike. The child shows no fear of the parent and, upon questioning, confirms the parent's version of the events. The staff reports the injury as a possible child abuse case.

3. You are a nursing student on a pediatrics rotation within the hospital and you notice that the neighbor of your parents has been admitted to the surgery unit. During your lunch break you review her record before you drop in to see her.

4. You are a technical nurse just completing postop care of a young woman who is a fellow church member and who has just had an abortion. You are very concerned for the young woman and decide to confide this information to your minister.

5. A young man who lives in the same housing complex that you do comes into the hospital's clinical laboratory for tests and is confirmed as being HIV positive. As the manager of that laboratory, you feel it a duty to tell the manager of the housing complex that, in fact, the person in Unit Five has an infectious disease.

6. You are a respiratory therapist, and your patient states that she would like to tell you something but only if you would hold it in strictest confidence. She then relates to you that she is very depressed and is thinking about taking her own life once she is discharged from the hospital. You relate this information to the attending physician.

7. You are a medical records technician and are in the department when two men come in and flash badges indicating that they are from the FBI and need to see the Hiram Jones record as a matter of national security. You cooperate and allow them access to the files.

8. In the course of caring for a patient, a bus driver, the physician notes that she is at risk for having a heart attack and recommends that she cease driving as she may be placing the children at risk. The driver asks that the physician not notify the school district as it would put her at risk of losing her job. The physician notifies the district.

9. During the course of a patient evaluation, you find that the family has incest problems. You recommend the notification of the police.

B. In the article, "Giving the Patient His Medical Record," the authors propose the following:[10]

> We propose that legislation be passed to require that complete and unexpurgated copy of all medical records, both inpatient and outpatient, be issued routinely and automatically to patients as soon as the services provided are recorded. The legislation should also require that physician and hospital qualifications and charges be recorded. Hospital records should be available regularly to patients on the ward, and copies sent to them upon termination of hospitalization.

In this exercise, first list four positive consequences that you think would come from such a law (for example, "Better communication between health care providers and patients") and then list four potential negative consequences (for example, "Increased litigation").

C. You are a student radiographer and are assigned to the surgery suite to assist another technician performing an X ray during a surgical procedure. You gown up, assist, and are present during much of the surgery that was being performed on Mrs. Jones by Dr. Smith.

Later the next day you are in Mrs. Jones's room and you comment that her choice of Dr. Smith was excellent in that he is a fine surgeon. "Dr. Smith?" she replies, "My physician was Dr. Goodhand! Call my lawyer!"

Have you breached confidentiality? In that it caused the hospital and physicians to be involved in a lawsuit, were you in error?

D. A couple comes into the emergency room, she complaining of vaginal discharge and pelvic pain and the husband of a urethral discharge. The tests done on the husband prove positive for gonorrhea and he adamantly demands that you keep this information from his wife. Her tests will not become available for two days. Should you tell the wife or maintain the confidentiality of the husband?

E. As the pharmacist of the local community pharmacy, you have been filling prescriptions for Mrs. Arthur for several years. She has an extensive medication profile that suggests that she has several chronic illnesses, including a psychiatric disorder. In her dealings with you there has been nothing that indicated an inability to make competent decisions or to authorize appropriate treatment decisions. One day her husband Bob comes into the pharmacy and requests that you give him a copy of his wife's medication profile. He indicates that he wants to be sure that his wife is receiving the correct medications and was being compliant in taking the drugs as prescribed.

For this problem we will use the RESOLVEDD method of problem solving developed by Dr. Raymond Pfeiffer. The steps of the process are:[11]

(R) Review facts involved.
> What are the relevant facts of the case?
> Who, if anyone, is at fault?
> How did the situation come about?
> Who is charged with making the decision?

(E) Estimate of the problem or conflict involved in case.
> What options do you have?
> What difficulties are presented by the case?
> What is the major ethical dilemma involved?

(S) State the solutions with initial credibility.
> Group the options into a small number of potential choices.

(O) Examine the Outcomes of the solutions.
> What are the significant possible outcomes that will result from following each of the potential solutions?

(L) Likely impact on those involved.
> In what way are those involved hurt or helped by the solutions?

(V) Values upheld/compromised.
> Which of the basic values are upheld or sacrificed by the solutions?

(E) Evaluation and refining of solution and weighing values.
> Which solution seems to have the best consequences for the individuals involved and sacrifices the least principles?

(D) Decision arrived at, clarified, and shown to implement equal consideration of interest.
> Decide how the decision will be carried out, and explain why this was the best of the possible solutions.

(D) Defense of that decision against objections to its main weaknesses.
> What are the major weaknesses of the decision?
> What are the best answers to objections based on the weaknesses?

Take each step as a separate exercise and work the problem through.

REFERENCES AND SUGGESTED READINGS

1. *Housh v. Peth,* 165 Ohio St 35, 133 NE 2d 340 (1956).
2. California Supreme Court; July 1, 1976, California Reporter 14.
3. Colorado Society of Clinical Specialists in Psychiatric Nursing, "Ethical Guidelines for Confidentiality," *Journal of Psychosocial Nursing* 28, no. 3 (1990): 43–44.

4. Sissela Bok, *Secrets: On the Ethics of Concealment and Revelation* (New York: Vintage Books, 1983).

5. Marc D. Hiller, "Computers, Medical Records, and the Right to Privacy." *Journal of Health Politics, Policy and Law* 6, no. 3 (Fall 1981): 463–487.

6. William Hafferty, "Whose Files Are They Anyway?" *Modern Maturity* (April-May 1991): 70.

7. Mark Siegler, "Confidentiality in Medicine—A Decrepit Concept," *New England Journal of Medicine* 307 (1982): 1518–1521.

8. Ill Ann Stat ch. 23 2054 (Smith-Hurd Supp. 1983-1984).

9. W. H. Roach, S. N. Chernoff and C. L. Esley, *Medical Records and the Law* (Rockville, MD: Aspen Publications, 1985).

10. Bud Shenkin and David Warner, "Giving the Patient His Medical Record: A Proposal to Improve the System," *New England Journal of Medicine* 289/13 (September 27, 1973): 688–699.

11. Raymond Pfeiffer and Ralph Fosberg, *Ethics on the Job* (Belmont, CA: Wadsworth Publishing Company, 1993).

—————— C H A P T E R 6 ——————

Aids and Health Care Practice

Instructional Goal

The major instructional goal for this chapter is to gain an understanding of the nature of the AIDS epidemic and to examine selected ethical problems associated with this crisis.

Instructional Objectives

At the end of this chapter the reader should understand and be able to:

1. Discuss the nature of the disease process of AIDS, and how it is acquired.
2. List the major infection control methods that have been used to bring the epidemic under control.
3. Explain how "universal precautions" have reduced the risk of infection for health care providers and what place they play in affirming a duty to treat.
4. List the high-risk behaviors associated with the spread of this disease.
5. List the reasons why confidentiality is perhaps more important for this patient group than for others we treat.
6. Write a rationale for the "duty to treat" this patient group.
7. List the conditions under which the moral duty to treat would cease to be a duty but only a moral option.
8. Write a series of guidelines that would provide the patient protection from AIDS-infected health care providers.
9. Provide rationales for the decisions both to tell and not tell health care providers the HIV status of the patients they care for.

Glossary

AIDS: Acquired Immune Deficiency Syndrome is generally accepted as a collection of specific, life-threatening, opportunistic infections that result from an underlying immune deficiency.

High-Risk Behaviors: A series of behaviors that are associated with the spread of AIDS infections.

Moral Duty: An act or course of action that is required by one on the basis of moral position.

Moral Option: The power or right to choose among several alternatives on the basis of a moral question.

"Safe Sex": A series of practices that are designed to allow for sexual contact that does not spread the AIDS virus. The most important aspect of these practices is the use of condoms.

Universal Precautions: Techniques adopted by health care providers that provide a barrier for acquiring AIDS. These are protective measures against contamination by blood or body secretions.

ETHICAL ISSUES OF AIDS

I was infected by Dr. Acer in 1987. My life has been sheer hell except for the good times and closeness with my family and my enjoyment for life and nature. AIDS has slowly destroyed me. Unless a cure is found, I will be another one of your statistics soon.

Who do I blame? Do I blame myself? I sure don't. I never used IV drugs, never slept with anyone, and never had a blood transfusion. I blame Dr. Acer and every single one of you bastards . . . anyone who knew Dr. Acer was infected . . . and stood by not doing a damn thing about it.[1]

Kimberly Bergalis

Early in the decade of the 1980s, health care practitioners within our major cities began to report patients with overwhelming and unusual opportunistic infections. These patients, usually young white males, presented with conditions thought to be rare and normally seen only in severely debilitated individuals or in textbooks. Relatively rare entities such as candidiasis of the esophagus, extrapulmonary cryptococcosis, Kaposi's sarcoma affecting a patient less than 60 years of age, progressive multifocal leukoencephalopathy, and pneumocystitis carinii became indicator diseases for what later became known as "Acquired Immunodeficiency Syndrome" or **AIDS.** Human Immunodeficiency Virus (HIV), which causes AIDS, is transmitted through sexual contact, exposure to infected blood or blood components, and perinatally from mothers to infants. While the HIV virus has been isolated from blood, vaginal secretions, semen, breast milk, saliva, tears, and cerebrospinal fluid, epidemiological evidence has implicated only blood, semen, vaginal secretions, and possibly breast milk in transmission. Table 6–1 lists the common transmission routes for the virus and its distribution by race and sex.[2]

AIDS evidently began as a mutant virus that was picked up from a species of African monkey and transferred to humans by way of bites. It was then transmitted among the African populations via direct mucous-to-mucous contact, through semen and perhaps blood exchange. From Africa, the disease spread to Haiti, and was later carried to the United States, probably by homosexual males. The heterosexual population became infected as blood supplies became contaminated and as a result of intravenous drug use and the sharing of contaminated needles. Female sexual partners of those infected through contaminated blood or needles contracted the disease through semen and spread the disease to other partners and perinatally to their infants. By 1990, it was estimated that over three million individuals were infected and that at least 20 percent of these would develop symptoms of the condition and die within the first half of this decade.

INFECTION CONTROL METHODS

As with other epidemics, the has Center for Disease Control sought to control the disease by breaking the chain of events causing the spread of the infection. This can be done in several ways such as decreasing the susceptibility of hosts; eliminating the source of the organisms; and interrupting the mode of transmission. Although some positive reports have come from researchers seeking a vaccine to decrease the susceptibility of individuals to the HIV virus, no current vaccine exists, and most researchers believe that it will be years before a safe and effective vaccine is devel-

TABLE 6–1
Reported Cases of AIDS in the United States, 1990

Category	Number	Percent
Sex		
Male	38,082	88
Female	5,257	12
Race		
Black	13,186	30
White	22,342	53
Hispanic	7,322	17
Transmission Category		
Men having sex with men	22,738	55
Injecting drugs	10,018	23
Heterosexual contact	2,711	06
Other	4,252	10
Unknown/unreported	2,620	06

oped. The major efforts toward eliminating the source of the infection have been through an active educational program, legal notification requirements, and special techniques in providing barriers at the point of direct and indirect contact. Between May 26 and June 30, 1988, the U.S.Department of Health and Human Services distributed over 107 million copies of the brochure "Understanding AIDS." With this mailing the government attempted to contact virtually every home and residential post office box regarding this public health problem.

The efforts directed toward breaking the chain of infection through special techniques to reduce the spread of infection in the general public has taken many forms. These range from the rather controversial methods such as clean needle exchange programs for IV drug users and provision of free condoms for high school students, to those less controversial such as screening prospective blood donors for high-risk behaviors, increased testing of blood supplies, and the promotion of "**safe sex**" or abstinence in high-risk situations. Recent studies in regard to the use of condoms for safe sex have indicated that perhaps the safety is more illusionary than real. In married couples in which one partner was HIV infected and condoms were used, 10 percent of the healthy became infected within two years.[3] The Health and Human Services brochure listing of both safe and **high-risk behaviors** is found in Figure 6–1.[4]

In their writings, Milliken and Greenblat[5] have suggested several specific criteria for an ethical social policy toward control of this epidemic. It was felt that only the adoption of such criteria would insure the acceptance by the citizenry, which is a basic requisite for successful policy.

1. Methods selected must be efficacious and appropriate to the stated goals.
2. The goals selected must be ethical, and equal consideration of interest must be central to processes.

Risky Behaviors
- Sharing Drug Needles and Syringes
- Anal Sex, With or Without a Condom
- Vaginal or Oral Sex With Someone Who Shoots Drugs or Engages in Anal Sex
- Sex With Someone You Don't Know Well (a pickup or prostitute) or With Someone You Know Has Several Sex Partners.
- Unprotected Sex (without a condom) with an infected person.

Safe Behaviors
- Not Having Sex
- Sex With One Mutually Faithful, Uninfected Partner
- Not Shooting Drugs

FIGURE 6–1 High-Risk and Safe Behaviors

3. Implementation of the policy must avoid discrimination and be justly administered

4. Harm to society or its subgroups that may result from the proposed policies must be identified and clearly understood.

5. The balance between harms and benefits must weigh heavily toward benefits.

OCCUPATIONAL RISK

In the hospital setting, efforts to protect health care workers and their patients have taken the form of adopting **Universal Precautions.** Figure 6–2 outlines the guidelines provided by the Occupational Safety and Health Administration (OSHA). In that medical history and examination cannot reliably identify all patients infected with HIV or other blood-borne pathogens such as hepatitis B, universal precautions have been recommended for all patients. This is especially critical for such practitioners as nurses, respiratory care specialists, and clinical laboratory technicians, as their work brings them into medical situations where contact with blood is common and the infection status of the patient is often unknown.[6]

In that great numbers of health care workers did not contract the disease in the early 1980s, it has become evident that the transmission modes for HIV are rather specific. The virus is a rather fragile entity, and there is little risk for practitioners who practice universal precautions and are otherwise not involved in high-risk behaviors.[7] One tragic exception to HIV infection being related to high-risk behaviors are the hemophiliac patients who acquired the disease in great numbers as a result of initial poor-quality testing of needed blood products used in their treat-

---

1. Wear Gloves when it is likely that hands will be in contact with body substances (blood, urine, feces, wound drainage, oral secretions, sputum, vomitus).

2. Protect clothing with a plastic apron or wear a gown when it is likely that clothing will be soiled with body substances.

3. Wear masks and or eye protection when it is likely that eyes, and or mucous membranes will be splashed with body substances (example: when suctioning a patient with copious secretions)

4. Wash hands often and well, paying particular attention to fingernails and the area between the fingers.

5. Discard uncapped needle/syringe units and sharps in puncture-resistant containers.

6. If unanticipated contact with body substances occurs, wash as soon as possible (hand washing, face washing, etc. as appropriate).

7. Use gloves to wipe up after all blood spills and disinfect using one part bleach to ten parts water.

FIGURE 6–2 Occupational Safety and Health Administration Guidelines, 1991 (Universal Precautions)

TABLE 6–2
CDC Data as of March 31, 1991, Listing Reported
AIDS Cases Among Health Care Providers

Profession	AIDS Cases
Nurses	1,358
Health Aides	1,101
Technicians	941
Physicians	703
Paramedics	116
Therapists	319
Dentists and hygienists	171
Surgeons	47
Miscellaneous health workers	1,680
Total	6,436

ment. Table 6–2 gives a listing of all reported cases of AIDS in health care workers since the epidemic began in the early 1980s. The vast majority of these cases were infections acquired outside the patient/provider relationship, so it is difficult to determine the risk for health care providers. Obviously, much depends on the nature of your duties: While the office worker is assuming virtually no risk, those involved in invasive procedures, emergency care, and childbirth are another matter. It is estimated that surgeons cut a glove during one in four procedures, and cut their own skin in one in forty. Of the million cases of HIV infections in the United States, by 1991 only the five involved with the Florida dentist, Dr. Acer, are known to have been infected by health care providers. As of 1991, there appear to have been forty health care providers who had contracted the disease from patients.[8] Of these, 27 were infected through needle sticks and six were caused by blood splashes into the eyes, mouth, or nose.

ETHICAL ISSUES AND THE AIDS EPIDEMIC

AIDS is a devastating epidemic with the potential for killing all who become infected. Although the risk of acquiring a hepatitis B infection is far higher, the deadly consequences of getting AIDS have made this disease a major ethical issue. In recent years, the population affected by the disease has extended into all groups, so that it is best not described by high-risk groups but rather by high-risk behaviors. The economic implications of AIDS is staggering. When one considers personal medical costs, direct costs of research, and indirect costs such as education, screening, and potential productivity losses, the disease carries a yearly price tag of over 66 billion dollars. The economic implication of these numbers is overwhelming when you consider the already overburdened health care system. Added to these tangible costs is another set of values that defy fiscal analysis—the loss of hopes, and dreams, and potential of its victims. What is the cost of these losses, when young people are handicapped during the time of their lives when they are at the peak of their productive work and childbearing years? One real problem with solving the AIDS dilemma is that many Americans appear to be experiencing a great deal of both fear and denial concerning their own risk of acquiring AIDS, and many have rationalized the continuation of lifestyles that place them at risk.[9]

The ethical problems associated with this disease are many and cut to the very heart of what it means to be a health care practitioner. The fact that AIDS has no known cure nor preventive vaccine makes it a disease that has caused the rethinking of basic fundamental issues. Do health care practitioners have a duty to treat? In a health care system already overburdened with the costs of health care, what resources should be allocated to a group of patients with a terminal disease? How much access to expensive technologies should terminal patients have? What is an acceptable risk for health care professionals? Should the patient be warned if the health care practitioner is HIV positive? Should the practitioner be warned if the patient is HIV positive? Should infected practitioners be allowed to continue practice? What is the meaning of confidentiality when it comes to AIDS, and who should be told?

DUTY TO TREAT

How much risk is acceptable for health care practitioners? Although much of the media have been directed toward patients who have been infected with the HIV virus by health care practitioners, the truth is that it is far more likely that the practitioner will be infected by the patient than the other way around.[10] A 1987 study showed that 1,875 adults with AIDS, for whom occupational information was available, reported being employed in a health care setting. In comparison, 6.8 millions persons, representing about 5.6 percent of the population of the United States labor force were employed in the health services. Of the health care providers reporting infection, 95 percent of these have been reported to exhibit high-risk behaviors; for the remaining 5 percent the means of HIV acquisition was undetermined. Health care workers were significantly more likely than other workers to have an undetermined risk of acquiring AIDS (5 percent versus 3 percent, respectively). Health care workers who have contracted the disease have included direct patient care groups such as physicians, dentists, nurses, nursing assistants, clinical laboratory technicians and therapists, but also groups such as housekeeping and maintenance, which usually do not have direct patient contact.

Although of great concern due to the tragic consequences of infection, the risk to health care practitioners seem to be very rare.[11] The use of universal precautions on all patients should provide an effective barrier and reduce the risk to an acceptable level. It would seem, then, that the limited risk to the practitioner would not provide a suitable rationale to refuse to treat patients with known HIV infections. In practice, it is probably not the known HIV infected patient who is most likely to spread the disease to health care workers. Figure 6–3 lists the recommended guidelines for practice in an epidemic as provided by the Health and Public Policy Committee of the American College of Physicians and the Infectious Disease

- To provide service consistent with skills
- To obtain skills if needed by patient population as consistent with scope of practice
- To provide accurate and Up-to-date information
- To promote the patient's best interest regardless of personal feelings toward patient or their disease entity[8]

FIGURE 6-3 Professional Duties in an Epidemic

Society of America. These guidelines find their basis in many of the health providers' codes of ethics, as example of which the nursing code for the care of victims of communicable disease calls for the "provision of services with respect for human dignity and the uniqueness of the client unrestricted by considerations of social or economical status, personal attributes, or the nature of the health problem." Nurses and allied health practitioners, then, have a duty to provide care commensurate with their scope of practice. Should the practitioner feel unsure in regard to universal precautions, there is an implicit duty to obtain the needed skills and to keep updated on all available information. Ignorance in this case might provide a short-term rationale for refusing to treat a patient with AIDS, but once the practitioner is trained in universal precautions, this would no longer provide a legitimate excuse. Western culture and health care practice provide historical precedence for the obligation to treat persons regardless of their social status, political affiliation, or even whether they be enemy or friend. The Good Samaritan ethic endorsed by our culture also provides strong ethical precedence for coming to the aid of those in danger or in need of help. This ethic of assistance does not, however, require that the rescuer take unacceptable risks in the process. For example, the nonswimmer is not expected to jump into the pool to save a drowning victim, for clearly this would not be in the interest of the victim or the potential rescuer.

What, then, does our culture require of us in regard to the AIDS patients? While we are not required to risk our lives in futile and perhaps dangerous gestures, under most situations that is not what we face with this patient group. While the potential for contracting AIDS within the workplace is a significant concern, it has occurred on an exceedingly infrequent basis. So this concern would not, in general, represent an acceptable rationale for refusing to treat but would create an obligation on the part of all health care workers to take appropriate protective actions.

The ANA Committee on Ethics offers some useful guidelines regarding the decision as to whether the practitioner has a moral duty to treat or whether the decision is left as a moral option. The four fundamental criteria are:[12]

1. The patient is at significant risk of harm, loss, or damage if the practitioner does not assist.
2. The practitioner's intervention or care is directly relevant to preventing harm.
3. The practitioner's care will probably prevent harm, loss, or damage to the patient.
4. The benefit the patient will gain outweighs any harm the practitioner might incur and does not present more than a minimal risk to the health care provider.

If the practitioner can answer yes to all four criteria, it would seem that a moral duty to treat would exist under the principle of beneficence. If, however, the circumstances place the practitioner in such a position that all criteria could not be answered with yes, then the decision to treat would become a moral option rather than a duty. An example of this might be an answer of no for the crucial fourth criterion, in a case where the practitioner finds a patient bleeding from the mouth, in respiratory failure and requiring CPR. Assuming that no masks or airways were in place, the decision to perform mouth-to-mouth resuscitation would not be mandated by duty.

Most health provider codes of ethics give a clear directive in regard to the treatment of patients regardless of their disease status. These moral directives have often been ignored, and certain health care providers have refused to treat HIV infected patients. In order to overcome this reluctance to treat this patient group, the government moved to include those infected with AIDS under the federal legislation barring discriminatory practices. This patient group is now afforded protection of Section 504 of the Rehabilitation Act of 1973. HIV serostatus and AIDS are now considered handicapping conditions covered under federal legislation prohibiting discriminatory practices. The failure to treat is no longer only a moral issue but also has potential legal consequences.[13]

CONFIDENTIALITY IN AN AGE OF AIDS

What I may see or hear in the course of the treatment or even outside of the treatment in regard to the life of men, which on no account one must spread abroad, I will keep to myself holding such things shameful to be noised about.

Hippocratic Oath

Confidentiality seems based on at least three foundations:(1)the duty-oriented acceptance of a personal right of self-determination, which requires the control over privacy and personal information;(2)the utilitarian view that if confidentiality were commonly breached, the patients would be deterred in seeking medical assistance for problems with sensitive or personal aspects; and (3)the long-held, virtue-oriented belief among health care providers that a special relationship exists between practitioner and client that calls for the tacit agreement of confidentiality and mutual trust.

It would seem that the first two of these foundations have a special importance when considering the AIDS epidemic. The nature of the illness and the recognition of its association with high-risk populations—such as homosexuals, drug users, and prostitutes—creates an enhanced danger of harm should private information be revealed beyond appropriate circles of care. Discrimination in housing, insurance, and employment, and even physical harm are very real outcomes of breaches of this patient group's confidentiality. Although rarely talked about in the press or in the national call for the screening of health care workers for AIDS, these same potential results from a breach in confidentiality must be considered equally in regard to the

HIV status of health care providers. Given the potential for personal harm, it is not hard to see that dedication to confidentiality is critical if this patient group is to be forthcoming in providing health care providers with the information necessary to contain the epidemic and provide adequate care. Because AIDS is universally fatal, protection of the uninfected must take precedence over other concerns, and those who are vulnerable must be warned. Unlike other infectious diseases, AIDS is also associated with a form of dementia as a result of which the infected individual may feel vindictive and intentionally try to transmit the virus.

When considering AIDS cases, the principle of confidentiality must be balanced with our obligations to provide appropriate disease control within the community and to protect vulnerable populations. Should a health care worker in the emergency department or an emergency medical technician (EMT) be notified that a patient who came into their care and whose bleeding they controlled was later confirmed to be HIV positive? In that all practitioners at this level should practice universal precautions for all patients—and understanding that, if practiced, these precautions reduce the vulnerability to a negligible risk—at first glance the answer would seem to be no. If the risk was minimal, and the practitioners were not vulnerable, confidentiality should not be broken. Stated differently, as autonomous moral agents who have accepted the role of health care provider, the practitioners have a duty to protect themselves in these cases, and if protected they would not be a particularly vulnerable population. Yet, on second consideration, anyone who has practiced in these situations knows that they are often less controlled than one might wish. The EMT reaching into the car to remove the bleeding patient often tears the gloves that are to provide the barrier; the emergency room worker is subject to needle or sharps sticks and barrier loss. While finding out after the fact that the patient was HIV positive might not be of use in preventing the health care provider from contracting the disease, it might provide essential information in regard to the need for testing, and could possibly save the family or other contacts of the health care provider. It is for these reasons that special categories of health care workers who are subject to direct body fluid contact have a right to know about the HIV status of their patients.

Recent surveys among practitioners show a general belief that those who are directly working with AIDS patients should be informed of their diagnosis. This information is not so much to allow practitioners to minimize personal risk as it is a fact that universal precautions are expected for all patients. The need to know has more to do with the professional tasks at hand, as it is difficult to provide adequate care without an accurate diagnosis. It is hard to imagine that a physician would feel comfortable treating a patient for whom someone else has decided that he or she should not be informed of the correct diagnosis. The level of professionalism of allied health practitioners and nurses would seem to make it reasonable that, indeed, they also need to know the diagnosis of the patients they treat. HIV positive status and the diagnosis of AIDS should be treated as any other disease; it should be part of the medical record. At the same time, if this were to be the policy of hospitals and clinics, it then becomes far more important that the charts be stored in a safe place so that patient confidentiality can be assured.

THE INFECTED HEALTH CARE PROVIDER

Public sentiment has long favored a policy of requiring health care providers to inform their patients if they have AIDS or a positive HIV status. A Gallup poll taken for *Newsweek* magazine found that 94 percent of Americans believe health care providers should be required to tell their patients if they are infected with the AIDS virus. Figure 6–4 indicates the types of health care workers who citizens feel should be required to relate their HIV status. A majority of those polled (65 percent) stated that they would discontinue all treatment if they discovered their physician was infected with the virus. This sentiment was brought forward even more strongly after the Center for Disease Control released a report that at least five individuals had been infected by Dr. David Acer, the Florida dentist mentioned earlier. It is suspected that the transmissions were caused by direct blood-to-blood contact. These cases were popularized in the media by the focus on Kimberly Bergalis, who won a one-million-dollar settlement from the dentist's insurance carrier and became a leader in a right-to-know movement directed toward forcing health care providers to tell their patients of their disease status.[14]

The Acer case caused a national panic among citizens as well as calls for mass screening of all practitioners. A lopsided majority vote occurred in favor of a bill sponsored by Senator Jesse Helms, of North Carolina, that would have imposed jail sentences on HIV positive health care providers who performed invasive procedures without first warning patients of their condition.

The Center for Disease Control estimates that the chance for transmission of the HIV virus by an infected surgeon to a patient is about one in 41,600 to 416,000 surgical procedures. This places the risk much lower than that of driving cars, or smoking cigarettes or even from dying from the anesthesia used for the surgery.[15] The case of *Behringer v. Medical Center,* at Princeton, New Jersey, dealt with an HIV infected surgeon who was allowed to practice. Upon finding out that the staff member was infected, the hospital allowed the physician to continue practice but limited his performance to procedures that posed no risk for HIV transmission. They also required that the physician obtain a written informed consent before performing any invasive procedure. The court based this decision on the ethical principles of beneficence/nonmaleficence as well as the conviction that patients themselves should have the final decision-making role in regard to whether they are willing to be treated by an infected practitioner.

Listing the types of health care providers that citizens believe should be required to tell patients of they are infected by the AIDS virus

95% - Surgeons
94% - All Physicians
94% - All Dentists
90% - All Health Care Workers

FIGURE 6–4 *Newsweek* Poll June 1991

The decision on how infected practitioners are to be treated in these cases seems to have been left up to the individual states, so long as their guidelines are at least equal to those promulgated by the Center for Disease Control.[16] At this time, of those states that have complied with the call for guidelines most have not required mandatory testing for health care workers nor have they required that practitioners limit their practice. The decision not to require mandatory testing seems to have been made on the basis of high cost and low effectiveness. While mandatory testing of all health care workers would seem to be a good solution, unfortunately it is ineffective because there can be a six-month lag between infection and the development of antibodies that can be identified in the test. Mandatory testing seems to offer more of an illusion of security than real substance. These tests also provide a certain level of false positives, which have the potential of destroying a practitioner's career. Most health care providers feel that rigorously enforced infection control methods would be more useful in protecting patients and providers than would mandatory testing.

Rather than requiring immediate cessation of practice or the limiting of practice to noninvasive techniques, the Center for Disease Control has recommended that expert review panels be set up to decide on a case-by-case basis whether seropositive health care workers should continue to perform invasive procedures.[8] The practitioner is required to communicate the positive HIV status to the health department, which is then charged with setting up an individual review of cases and a monitoring process. The review process would call for counseling of the infected practitioner and would rate the danger to patients. If it was decided that the infected practitioner posed a threat to patients he would be advised to notify all affiliated institutions of his status. In that certain HIV positive patients experience a period of dementia as part of their disease process, strict practice limitations and close monitoring seem appropriate. There are indications that the Florida dentist who infected Bergalis and others did so on purpose, perhaps as a result of paranoia brought on by his disease.

SUMMARY

Acquired Immune Deficiency Syndrome (AIDS) continues to grow as a worldwide epidemic. The disease, which at one time was centered within certain high-risk groups, has now spread into all segments of the population. The study of high-risk groups is no longer the best way to identify those at risk for the disease; rather, risk should be measured through the observance of certain high-risk behaviors. Due to the frightening consequences of the disease and its relative newness, the public has reacted very negatively toward those infected. Victims of the disease have been stigmatized, exposed to humiliation, and have experienced loss of work, insurance, and housing. The issue of confidentiality and the attempt to sustain a level of privacy beyond that provided for other diseases often create problems for the patient and the health care provider. AIDS is the only disease about which there is any question as to whether health care providers should be told the diagnosis of their patients. In some sense, the confidentiality and privacy provided the Florida dentist were a major cause of the tragic death of Kimberly Bergalis. Ethical issues involved with this disease include confidentiality, the duty to treat infected individuals, the need for universal screening, the duty of infected health care providers to warn patients, and the need for equitable distribution of medical care and research dollars. It is clear that the resources that will be needed to care for these patients threaten to overwhelm an already burdened health care delivery system.

None of these issues has yet been satisfactorily addressed. How we finally address and resolve these problems will speak either well or ill of the ethical foundations of the American health care system. Because of the scope of the ethical problems associated with the AIDS epidemic, our actions in response to it will leave either a proud or a shameful heritage for future health care providers.

CLARIFICATION EXERCISES

A. In the following scenarios, determine the correct provider response. Justify your answer.
   1. If the nurse attending the patient were herself immune suppressed, would this be enough to move the duty to treat an HIV infected patient to the moral option of treating or not treating?
   2. You are a respiratory therapist and have been assigned to a floor unit. You find that your department head has decided to reuse patient suction traps in order to save money. This is a breach of universal precautions. What should your response be?
   3. As an EMT, you punctured your gloves while removing an auto accident victim from her car. In this case, would you have a legitimate right to know her HIV status?
   4. You are a physical therapist and have been seeing Mr. Jones for months as a result of a referral from Dr. Smith. Over this time period, your relationship has grown until the patient has a better relationship with you than with his physician. One day he tells you that he is HIV positive and asks that you not tell the Dr. Smith. What action do you take?
   5. You are a dental hygienist and have found out that you are pregnant. Is this a rationale for refusing to treat HIV infected patients?
   6. In that Dr. Acer has caused alarm among dental patients, your clinic has decided to advertise in the local paper that all your staff is "HIV free." Is this ethical?

B. Consider the following proposal and determine whether the idea has merit. Is it ethical? Does it protect the interests of society and the HIV positive individual? What are the negatives to such a policy?

If we assume that AIDS, in most cases, is contracted as the result of the performance of high-risk behaviors, generally, an individual with AIDS must share some responsibility for contracting the disease. Some important exceptions would be individuals who contract the disease from contaminated blood products or health care workers or patients who contract the disease as a result of medical care.

As a society, AIDS is going to require great expenditures of resources both in research and in providing care for those affected—as well as the terrible losses in human potential. Currently AIDS consumes as much of the research dollars as does heart disease and cancer.

Individual risk from contracting the disease could be somewhat lessened if affected individuals self-reported. If, for instance, one knew that a lover or fellow IV drug user was infected one could more easily avoid contracting the disease.

Would it be fair, given the great cost that society is going to have to bear and the fact that for the most part this disease is somewhat self-inflicted, to require HIV positive individuals to receive a small tattoo on the underarm identifying them as having the disease? The tattoo would be placed high on the underarm and would be very unobtrusive, but it could be checked for by lovers, fellow drug users, ambulance workers, and others who might need to know this information.

C. U.S. Public Health policy has been very restrictive in accepting blood from sexually active homosexual and bisexual men with multiple partners. Some gay activists have seen this as stigmatizing the gay community, which includes both infected and noninfected individuals. This appears to be a conflict between the right to give a gift and the right of the individual who receives the blood to know that the gift of blood is pure.

State your opinion in regard to the argument. Is there a compromise position that would be satisfactory to both groups?

REFERENCES AND SUGGESTED READING

1. *New York Times,* 22 June 1991:A5.
2. *Reported Cases of HIV Infection and AIDS in the United States, 1990, MMWR* 41, no. 15 (17 April 1992).
3. D. R. Mishell, "Contraception," *The New England Journal of Medicine,* 320 (1989): 777–787.
4. *Understanding AIDS,* HHS Publication no. (CDC) HHS-88-8404.
5. Nancy Milliken and Ruth Greenblatt, *Ethical Issues of the AIDS Epidemic* (Rockville, MD: An Apen Publication, 1988).
6. National Safety Council, *Bloodborne Pathogens* (Boston: Jones and Bartlett Publishers, 1993).
7. Deborah Henderson, *"HIV Infection: Risks to Health Care Workers and Infection Control," Nursing Clinics of North America* 23, no. 4 (December 1988): 767–775.
8. Donise Grady, *"Infected Healers," American Health (April 1991): 30–33.*
9. P. Glenn, L. Spronson, M., McCartney, and C., Yesalis, *"Attitudes Toward AIDS Among a Low Risk Group of Women, JOGNN Clinical Studies, 20, no. 5 (September/October 1990): 398–405.*
10. Bernard Lo and Robert Steinbrook, "Health Care Workers Infected with the Human Immunodeficiency Virus," *Journal of the American Medical Association 267, no. 8 (26 February 1992): 1100–1105.*
11. Health and Public Policy Committee, American College of Physicians, and the Infectious Disease Society of America, "Position Paper on Acquired Immunodeficiency Syndrome," *Annals of Internal Medicine* 104 (1986): 575–581.
12. American Nurses' Association, *Code for Nurses with Interpretitive Statements* (Kansas City Missouri: American Nurses Association, 1985).
13. Eileen Kolasa, "HIV vs. a Nurse's Right to Work" *RN* (January 1993): 63–66.
14. Thomas Witherspoon, "Florida Case Raises Ethical Concerns," *Registered Dental Hygiene Journal,* Dental Hygiene Association (January 1991): 52–53.
15. Debbie Beck, "Mandatory HIV Testing for Health Care Workers: Is It Ethical?" *Nursing Forum* 27, no. 4 (October 1992): 9–14.
16. Larissa A. Kuntz, "CDC Shifts Control," *RT Image* 6, no. 29 (20 July 1992).
17. L. Bernard and R. Steinbrook, "Health Care Workers Infected With the Human Immunodeficiency Virus," *JAMA* 267, no. 8 (26 February 1992): 1100–1105.

Withholding and Withdrawing Life Support

Instructional Goal

At the end of this chapter the reader will understand the various arguments used and the types of patients involved in the issues of withdrawing and withholding life support.

Instructional Objectives

At the end of this chapter the reader should understand and be able to:

1. Differentiate between "life" as defined in a biological or biographical sense.
2. State the necessity for redefining death beyond that of a loss of cardiac and pulmonary function, which in many circumstances can be sustained by modern technology.
3. Define the concept and criteria of brain death.
4. Outline the rationale for the proposal to redefine death with a neocortical definition.
5. Define PVS and state the characteristics of the syndrome.
6. Differentiate between the "best interest" and "substituted "judgment" standards as they relate to proxy decisions.
7. Define the difference between "ordinary and extraordinary care."
8. Outline the problems associated with the standard differentiations given for ordinary and extraordinary care.
9. Differentiate between the various lines of reasoning and arguments needed to decide the following types of cases in regard to withdrawing or withholding care:

      a. Persistent Vegetative State cases

      b. Profoundly Retarded Patient cases

      c. Baby Doe cases

      d. Informed nonconsent cases

10. Outline the arguments for personhood criteria and state how they could be used in withdrawing care determinations.

11. Define what is meant by the "Clear and Convincing Evidence" standard.

12. Explain the difference between the two major types of "Advanced Directives"—"Living Wills" and "Durable Power of Attorney."

13. Differentiate between active and passive euthanasia.

Glossary

Advanced Directives: Documents that relate to others your wishes should you lose the ability to relate these matters yourself.

Best-Interest Standard: A proxy decision-making standard where the guardian is directed to make the decision in the best interest of the individual. This is often used in cases where the individual was never in a position to make an autonomous decision.

Big Ethics: The ethics concerning those dramatic issues surrounding life and death. Little ethics concern the day by day issues such as confidentiality and veracity.

Biographical Life: Life described by events, relationships, memories, desires, and wishes. Life that is uniquely individual and human.

Biological Life: Life that separates the living from the nonliving, e.g., that separates plants from rocks. Life in this sense is not uniquely human but is that which we share with all other living things.

Brain Death: Irreversible cessation of all functions of the entire brain, including the brain stem. This is a totally unresponsive, irreversible state beyond coma.

Clear and Convincing Evidence Standard: Following the Nancy Cruzan case, the courts have asked for clear and convincing evidence of the individuals' wishes in regard to continuing or ceasing life support. This has created a new emphasis on the need for advanced directives.

Cognitive Sapient State: A condition in which the individual has the ability to reason.

DNR (Do Not Resuscitate) Orders: Those orders issued when a determination is made that the level of life that could be sustained following resuscitative efforts would be such that they would not be in the patient's best interest.

Durable Power of Attorney: A legal document that identifies another individual who is empowered to make decisions for you in your absence or inability to make your wishes known.

Euthanasia: Easy death, the concept of assisting another in dying.

Neocortical Death: Irreversible loss of high brain function, which allows personal capacity. Often patients who have lost neocortical function have lost the potential for all uniquely human aspects of life but still maintain vegetative function.

Ordinary and Extraordinary Care: A differentiation used to determine what level of care is required and the level that might be considered optional due to high costs, low effectiveness, or other criteria.

Parens Patria: Originates from the English common law, whereby the King had the authority to act as guardian for persons with legal disabilities. In the United States, the parens patria function belongs to the states.

Patient Self-Determination Act of 1990 (PSDA): Mandates that all health care providers receiving federal reimbursements for services provide information to each patient and offer the option of initiating an advanced directive.

Personhood: The individual state in which one is accepted as having the criterion of humanity.

PVS (Persistent Vegetative State): Characterized by a permanent eyes-open state of unconsciousness.

Quality of Life Issue: The question of whether the potential quality of an individual's life is the primary consideration regarding decisions involving resuscitation or other extraordinary measures.

Right-to-Die Movement: A group of individuals who subscribe to the concept that, along with the protected rights of life, liberty, and the pursuit of happiness, individuals have the right to decide when life should be ended.

Substituted-Judgment Standard: A proxy decision-making standard whereby the guardian is directed to make the decision compatible with the previous wishes of the individual.

BIOLOGICAL AND BIOGRAPHICAL LIFE

I cannot but have reverence for all that is called life. I cannot but avoid compassion for all that is called life. This is the beginning and foundation of morality. . . It is good to maintain and cherish life; it is evil to destroy and check life.

Albert Schweitzer[1]

Possibly . . . no contemporary superstition is so stupid and pernicious as the indiscriminate adoration of the word life, used without any definite meaning but effectively hiding the fact that life includes the most loathsome forms of disease and degradation. Sanity and wisdom consist not in the pursuit of life but in the pursuit of the good life. . .

Morris Cohen[2]

Of all the problems that can be considered **big ethics,**[3] none has caused the same level of moral anguish as that of withholding and withdrawing life-support systems. The attitudes and values expressed in the quote by Dr. Schweitzer are a positive affirmation of life, and it is often sentiments such as these that bring individuals to the practice of health care. Today, however, the practitioner is faced with the frustrating problem of available technology that allows for life extension but cannot restore the patient to a life free of pain and misery—or even, in some cases, to an awareness of the environment. This frustration often leads to a new attitude toward life, one that finds expression in statements like the one above by Morris Cohen. The practitioner's duty to respect life and preserve it where possible may at times come into direct conflict with the duty to alleviate pain and suffering. The Hippocratic Oath binds physicians to take upon themselves the duty to adopt practices that shall benefit the patients and protect them from hurt or wrong. What is to be done when the care we offer appears to have no value to the patient? What is to be done when the quality of life restored has a negative value, when life itself appears to be an added injury?

REDEFINING THE CONCEPT OF LIFE

It has been suggested that what is needed is a restatement of what is meant by the word "life." In the common usage of the term, we often mean two very different things. In one sense we use the word living to differentiate the things of our world into two basic categories, one of bugs, bushes, deer, and humans, which are considered living things, and the other of air, water, minerals, etc., which are nonliving things. With the question, "Is there life on other planets?" we are thinking of life in a biological sense. While, on the one hand, **biological life** is not uniquely human, we also separate the life of humans into a different category from the life we share with trees—the human life that is captured in weddings, events, relationships, etc., which can be termed biographical life. In the once-popular television program, *"This is Your Life,"* the sense is that of **biographical life.** It is our life events—our relationships, dreams, and expectations—that truly separate us from other life forms and make us uniquely human.

Anyone involved in the practice of critical care medicine can readily bring to mind patients who, due to injury, arrive in the ICU in a coma and are placed on life-support systems. If the brain damage is extensive, and the care is of high quality, some of these patients can survive in a **persistent vegetative state (PVS)** for months or even years. With current technology, we can often sustain life in a biological sense, but we cannot restore individuals to an awareness of themselves or others. In many cases, an individual may survive for years without gaining consciousness. The gravestone of Nancy Cruzan, as shown in Figure 7–1, indicates the level of ambiguity that is often felt in regard to the individual value of biological life.[4]

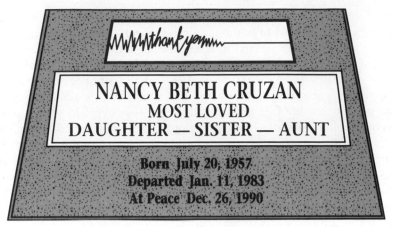

NANCY BETH CRUZAN
MOST LOVED
DAUGHTER — SISTER — AUNT

Born July 20, 1957
Departed Jan. 11, 1983
At Peace Dec. 26, 1990

FIGURE 7–1

The decision to preserve biological life at any cost leads to immense personal and social tragedies that consume individuals, human energies, and scarce resources—for no seeming good. The question, then, is what is to be done when all individual personality has irretrievably fled and all we can sustain is biological life?

BRAIN DEATH

One essential differentiation among patient types is between those who have suffered brain death and those who are in a persistent vegetative state (PVS). With the modern technology of respiratory and cardiac support, in certain cases of severe brain trauma we can keep the remainder of the body's cells alive for days and months with no brain activity being present. This has raised major problems in terms of the classic definition of death based on the loss of cardiac and pulmonary function. As a result of these technological changes, a majority of jurisdictions within our nation have accepted the concept of **brain death.** Figure 7–2 lists the criteria for brain death given by the Harvard Medical School Ad Hoc Committee.[5]

Brain death cases are often very problematic to families, as the patient appears to have natural warmth and color, the EKG may be in sinus rhythm, and the chest rises and falls with each cycle of the ventilator. Families view these as signs of life and need time to be brought to an understanding of the true condition. During this period of counseling, the practitioners will often broach the question of consent in order to arrange for the harvest of valuable organs for transplantation.

At these times, a natural shift occurs; nothing more can be done for the brain dead patient, who is deceased. The support of the family in this time of personal loss becomes the major concern of the health care practitioner. In a real sense the family become the patients with whom the health care practitioners are involved. Great care and sensitivity must be taken as equipment is removed. Often the devices are turned down slowly so that cardiac failure takes place to simulate death. The

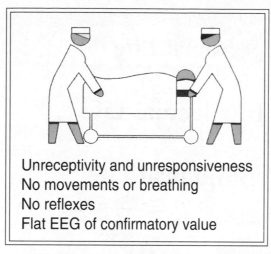

Unreceptivity and unresponsiveness
No movements or breathing
No reflexes
Flat EEG of confirmatory value

FIGURE 7–2 Brain Death Harvard Test

removal of the equipment, however, is not an act of "allowing to die," as, in fact, a corpse (as defined by brain death) cannot be thought to die. Out of respect to the families, or out of fear of legal issues, practitioners may delay the removal of life-sustaining equipment, but no consent is required for unhooking a ventilator from a dead body.

One interesting formulation of what constitutes death is an attempt by Thomas Furlow[6] to look at death not as an event but rather as a process of withdrawal (Figure 7–3). According to this model, the process of dying can be likened to three concentric circles. The outermost ring is made up of one's interpersonal relationships and is called the *Social Life*. Being outermost, this is the most vulnerable of the aspects of our being and usually is the first to die. The individual then withdraws to the middle circle which represents human *Intellectual Life*, that part of ourselves that separates us from the rest of the biological world. Consciousness and interaction, deriving from the highest level of the brain or the cerebrum, characterize this level. Once dying has claimed this region, biographical death has occurred and only the innermost ring is left—*biological life*, controlled largely by the brain stem. As we have said, this form of life is not uniquely human because it shares common features with nonhuman life forms. Loss of function in this region constitutes biological death. Some authorities have argued that the time is near when medicine will need to revise the definition of death beyond the "brain dead" criterion to include neocortical death[7]. A person would be considered dead by this criterion if only the higher brain centers, and not the entire brain, had lost function irreversibly. Under this criterion many patients in a persistent vegetative state who have the potential for years of vegetative life would be judged dead. However, some real problems are involved as patients have come back from a persistent vegetative state. In brain death, the body ceases to function once ventilatory support is discontinued. With PVS, the patient would continue to breathe once devices now considered ordinary care were removed. The adoption of this standard necessitates additional movement toward active euthanasia, for which, at present, we have no consensus.

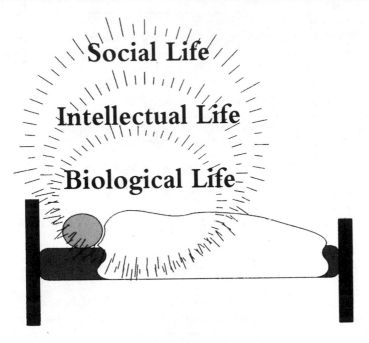

FIGURE 7-3

PERSISTENT VEGETATIVE STATES

In April 1975, a 21-year-old female, while with friends, ingested an undetermined amount of alcohol and tranquilizers. She was brought to the hospital in a coma, having suffered two periods of apnea (not breathing) lasting for at least 15 minutes. This resulted in brain damage with the diagnosis of PVS, in which she had no recognizable cognitive function. PVS is characterized by a permanent eyes-open state of unconsciousness. The patient is not comatose; she is awake but unaware. The eyes are often vacant and often the patient assumes a severely contracted body position. Clinically, PVS suggests the irreversible loss of all neocortical function. Generally, brain stem functions remain and patients can breathe on their own. They do not, however, match the criteria of brain death, inasmuch as they have elicitable reflexes, spontaneous respirations, and reactions to external stimuli. Recovery from a persistent vegetative state is rather remote. Using the guidelines of waiting three months in cases of PVS following cardiac arrest, six months for patients below 40 with head injuries, and 12 months for patients below 25 with head injuries, the chance of any sort of recovery is less than one in a thousand.

The 21-year-old patient remained in this state for a period of seven months, being sustained by a ventilator and feeding tubes. At this time, the physicians in the case indicated to the family that it was their opinion that there was no hope she would ever regain consciousness and that she would die if ventilatory support was removed. After hearing this grim prognosis, the family requested the ventilator be removed: It was their religious conviction that this was in keeping with God's will, and they felt that their daughter would not have wanted to live this way. However, in that the patient did not match the criteria for brain death, the physicians refused to remove the ventilator and the family took the matter to court.

The press exposure from this early case made Karen Ann Quinlan a name recognized by everyone and brought increased awareness of the need for a procedure whereby extraordinary care could be withdrawn from patients.[8]* In the lower court decision, the family was refused permission to have the ventilator removed. However, on appeal, the New Jersey Supreme Court overturned the lower court decision and appointed Karen's father as her guardian for purposes of discontinuing the ventilator. The court ruled that when an individual has no chance of recovering a **cognitive sapient state** the argument for the protection of life weakens and the individual's right to privacy may call for discontinuance of burdensome life support, as determined by a guardian. Karen's nurses, understanding that the court might grant the family permission to remove the ventilator, began to wean the patient from the device, so that when it was finally removed she continued to breathe. Karen remained in a persistent vegetative state for an additional ten years. In June 1985, she contracted acute pneumonia and died. Antibiotics that might have been used to continue her existence were not used.

During the additional decade of her life following her removal from the ventilator, Karen was sustained by feeding tubes and IV fluids. Had these been removed along with her ventilator, she would have died ten years earlier. The case of Karen Ann brings up many ethical problems in regard to not only removal of ventilators from patients with no chance of recovering but also what constitutes **ordinary and extraordinary care.**

ORDINARY AND EXTRAORDINARY CARE

It is generally held that one can ethically forgo extraordinary means of continuing life but is obliged to continue ordinary means of care. In the 1957 encyclical, "Prolongation of Life," by Pope Pius XII, this view was reaffirmed that in the prolongation of life "one was held to use only ordinary means—according to circumstances of persons, places, times, and culture—that is to say, means that do not involve any grave burden to oneself or another."[9] Although not binding as a statement of practice, the encyclical was important given that the source could be expected to be on the conservative side of the sanctity of life issue.

Questions regarding what constitutes ordinary and extraordinary care have generally resulted in classification of items such as oxygen, antibiotics and IV fluids listed as "ordinary," while ventilators, extracorporeal oxygenators, and dialysis devices are "extraordinary." This analysis has two basic problems, in that it does not take into consideration technological advancement or patient reference. For example, in the United States, we had a critical shortage of dialysis devices in the 1960s, and therefore the treatments were considered extraordinary. Today, through technological advancement and resource allocation, we have an adequate supply of equipment and kidney dialysis has become ordinary care. The second problem is the lack of patient reference. What might be extraordinary care for a 92-year-old with terminal cancer, might be considered ordinary for a 30-year-old post-appendectomy patient. A good example of lack of patient reference was the nasogastric feeding and IV fluids given to Karen Ann Quinlan. Under normal conditions, these are considered ordinary; however their continuance forced Quinlan to continue a life without personal value for another decade following the removal of the ventilator. In that the procedures offered no reasonable hope of benefit, perhaps they also were extraordinary care.

Figure 7–4 gives a formulation provided by Father Gerald Kelly, S.J, for ordinary and extraordinary care that allows for consideration of costs, pain, inconvenience, and potential benefit. Under this definition, the problems of technological change and patient reference are satisfied. Any form of care can be extraordinary if it offers no hope of benefit. Under this definition, IV fluids and nasogastric feedings would qualify as extraordinary care in patients with PVS as they offer no potential benefit.[10] With this line of reasoning, the focus is placed on the usefulness and burdensomeness of care rather than on any characteristic of the treatment itself. There are other scholars, however, who would argue that food and water are not in a real sense medical care at all but rather "the sort of care that all human beings owe each other" as a function of our common humanity.[11] The removal of food and water seems more causally related to the death of the patient, than just standing aside and allowing him or her to die.

PERSONHOOD

One rather controversial line of reasoning that seems appropriate for cases involving patients in a persistent vegetative state with no hope for recovery is the examination of the requirements of **personhood.** While we generally agree that human beings have certain rights and privileges, and that these rights are not extended to rocks, trees, or animals, what is the essential difference? What types of beings can be thought of as bearers of rights? What types of beings can be thought of as persons?

Ordinary Means are all medicines, treatments, and operations that offer a reasonable hope of benefit and which can be obtained without excessive expense, pain, or other inconvenience.

Extraordinary Means are all medicines, treatments, and operations that cannot be obtained or used without excessive expense, pain, or other inconvenience or which, if used, would not offer a reasonable hope of benefit.

FIGURE 7–4 Ordinary vs. Extraordinary Means

Philosophers such as Joseph Fletcher[12] and Joel Feinberg[13] have attempted to define characteristics that a being must possess in order to be considered a bearer of rights. Among the suggested criteria are:

1. One who could be said to have interests; a person for whom something can be said to be good for his or her own sake.

2. One who has cognitive awareness; a being of memories, expectations, and beliefs.

3. One who is capable of relationships. Interpersonal relationships seem to be at the very essence of what we idealize in truly being a person.

4. One who has a sense of futurity. How truly human is someone who cannot realize there is a time yet to come as well as a present? The words "What do you want to become" only makes sense in relation to a person.

If these criteria were accepted as being necessary for one to be considered a bearer of rights (a person), then patients in PVS do not meet the criteria. Whereas Karen Ann Quinlan, prior to her accident, may have had the right to vote, right to freedom of speech, etc., it becomes incomprehensible to consider her as a possessor of these rights once she irreversibly lost neocortical function. These patients cannot be thought of as being the kinds of beings for whom rights make sense—either the right to life or the right to die. Since the patient who has become irreversibly comatose is not one who can be thought of as having interests, nothing we do to them can run counter to their interests. In this sense, what we do or don't do is rather dependent upon the interests of others—society, family, health care practitioners—who can be considered bearers of rights. The patients themselves can be left out of the equation. Some have suggested that personhood should replace brain death as the legitimate criterion for death. For others, the personhood argument is a rather slippery slope that could allow some monstrous wrong to be perpetrated against a helpless minority in the future. The historical precedence of one group denying others the classification of personhood and then using this argument to justify slavery or sterilization rings frighteningly true and appalling. What can militate against such a philosophy is that the criterion being used for personhood is currently very basic. As long as the definitions remain at the level of self-awareness, no potential group of targeted and persecuted minorities could be excluded. Denying personhood to those with PSV does not say anything about them or suggest what it is that we might do to or for them; it just excludes them from the community of those who can be thought to bear rights.

It is clear that the reasoning involved in questions of personhood are of vital importance to the study of biomedical ethics. Most of the focus of ethical thought is the person, the being who bears personal rights and responsibilities. In the past, judgments in this regard have excluded such groups as women, blacks, and American Indians. Our current abortion debate is the most obvious situation in which we are searching for the definition of a human being. Many in our society hold that the fetus becomes a person with all the rights and privileges of such a being at the moment of conception; others hold that this status is delayed until viability. If you accept viability as the standard, then personhood is dependent upon technology inasmuch as a fetus is considered viable somewhere near the 24th week in the United States, but near 30 weeks in Ethiopia. With the utilization of artificial wombs in the future, personhood might be pushed back to a period near conception. Depending on where you place personhood along the scale of life, you draw very different ethical decisions. It is one thing to abort a piece of tissue (regardless of how remarkable) and quite another to abort a person.

ADVANCED DIRECTIVES

In 1983, at 25 years of age, Nancy Cruzan lost control of her car and was thrown into a ditch. Although she was resuscitated at the scene of the accident, she never regained consciousness. Like Karen Ann Quinlan, Nancy was diagnosed as being in PVS, and physicians estimated that she could live for another 30 years being supported by feeding tubes. In describing her condition, her father stated that "Since the accident, she has never had what we felt was a thought produced response to anything. We feel the most humane and kind thing we can do is to help her escape this limbo between life and death."[14] Given the prognosis, the family requested that the feeding tube be removed and Nancy be allowed to die. When the Missouri Rehabilitation Center refused the request, the family took the case to the lower courts, which ruled in their favor. This affirmation was overturned by the State Supreme Court on the basis that the state's greater duty to preserve life outweighed any right that the parents might have to refuse treatment for their daughter.

In December 1989, the Cruzan case became the first of the right-to-die cases to be heard by the Supreme Court of the United States. In its decision, the Court upheld the Missouri Supreme Court position that not even the family should make choices for an incompetent patient in the absence of "clear and convincing evidence" of the patients' wishes. In a five-four decision, the Court ruled that states do have these rights for the following reasons:[15]

- The state has a right to assert an unqualified interest in the preservation of human life.

- A choice between life and death is an extremely personal matter.

- Abuse can occur when incompetent patients don't have loved ones available to serve as surrogate decision makers.

- The state has a right to express an unqualified interest in the preservation of human life.[15]

To accommodate the **clear and convincing evidence standard** required by the court, three friends of Nancy came forward claiming to have had conversations with her prior to the accident in which she expressed the conviction that she would never want to live the life of a vegetable. As a result, the State of Missouri no longer opposed her parents in this action and the feeding tube was removed. Nancy Cruzan died shortly after the removal.

The call for clear and convincing evidence in regard to these cases has increased the interest in **advanced directives.** Following the example set by California in 1976, more than 40 states have passed some form of "living will" (Figure 7–5), "right-to-

I, _____ am of sound mind, and I voluntarily make this declaration.

I direct that life-sustaining procedures should be withheld or withdrawn if I have an illness, disease, or injury, or experience extreme mental deterioration, such that there is no reasonable expectation of recovering or regaining a meaningful life.

These life-sustaining procedures that may be withheld or withdrawn include, but are not limited to:

Cardiac resuscitation, ventilatory support, antibiotics, artificial feeding and hydration.

I further direct that treatment be limited to palliative measures only, even if they shorten my life.

Specific instructions:

A. Specific instructions regarding care I do want:

B. Specific instructions regarding care I do not want:

My family, the medical facility, any physicians, nurses, and other medical personnel involved in my care shall have no civil or criminal liability for following my wishes as expressed in this declaration.

I sign this document after careful consideration.

I understand its meaning and I accept its consequences.

Date:_____ Signed: _____

Address: _____

_____

This Declaration was signed in our presence. The declarant appears to be of sound mind and to be making this declaration voluntarily without duress, fraud or undue influence.

Signed by witness: _____

Signed by witness: _____

FIGURE 7–5 Living Will Statement

die" or "death-with-dignity" statute. There is, however, no uniformity in laws on living wills and surrogate decision makers. In some states, the advanced directives go into effect only if a patient is terminally ill and death is imminent. In others, the physician is given civil and criminal immunity from prosecution when he or she fails to honor the living will, when in his or her judgment continued treatment may be of benefit to the patient and if it is a good faith action based on medically valid reasons. In over 20 states the will is invalidated during pregnancy.

Due to the inconsistencies and limitations found in these statutes, many authorities recommend the use of **durable power of attorney** over a living will. This allows you to name someone as proxy, with the authority to make medical decisions on your behalf should you become incompetent and unable to make the decisions yourself. This form of legal arrangement seems to offer the greatest flexibility in making your wishes known after you have lost competency, as the proxy individual is in the position to react to changes in your situation. The Society for the Right to Die suggests the following reasons for establishing a durable power of attorney:[17]

1. To give or withhold consent to specific medical or surgical measures with reference to the principal's condition, prognosis, and known wishes regarding terminal care; to authorize appropriate end-of-life, including pain-relieving, procedures.
2. To grant releases to health care providers.
3. To employ and discharge health care providers.
4. To have access to and to disclose medical records and other personal information.
5. To resort to court, if necessary, to obtain court authorization regarding medical treatment decisions.
6. To expend or withhold funds necessary to carry out medical treatments.

According to a 1988 study by the American Medical Association, quoted in Newsweek July 1990, only 15 percent of our citizens had any form of advanced directive in place. Young people and the poor are the least likely to request and implement these forms. As is true with many social issues, the poor and poorly informed suffer the consequences of having the least protection. The **Patient Self-Determination Act of 1990 (PSDA),** shown in Figure 7–6, mandates that all certified hospitals, nursing facilities, home health care agencies, hospices, and HMOs receiving federal reimbursement under Medicare and Medicaid provide adult clients with information on living wills and other forms of advanced directives.[18] Although nurses and other health care providers will perform a vital service in the education of patients about advanced directives, they are prohibited from serving as witnesses to durable power of attorney directives, which involve the patients they serve.

Although the Supreme Court held to a narrow focus in the Nancy Cruzan case, several critical aspects were reinforced by the decision. First, the Court upheld the concept that competent individuals could refuse life-sustaining treatment. Second, it made no legal distinction between tube feeding and other life-sustaining measures. Food and water may be withheld when either of the two following conditions are met:[19]

1. The treatment is futile: In cases where all efforts to provide nutrition would be ineffective and cause pain, e.g., those patients where the cardiac status is such that any IV fluids would overload the heart.
2. No possibility of benefit: While it is most often reasonable practice to provide nutrition and hydration, in those cases where the family and caregivers agree that the practice offers no benefit, such as a PVS case, there should be no barrier to discontinuance.

Senator John Danforth (R-Mo.) drafted the PSDA as part of the Omnibus Reconciliation Act of 1990. PSDA was designed to support the autonomous decision-making authority of patients in regard to accepting or refusing specific medical interventions when admitted to healthcare facilities receiving federal reimbursements under Medicare or Medicaid. The legislation requires these facilities to:

A. Provide patients at the time of admissions with information concerning their right to accept or refuse medical interventions. The facilities are charged with providing information and assistance in the preparation of advanced directives.

B. The facilities will create and maintain written institutional policies in regard to patient rights. They will provide education for the staff, patients, and community concerning advanced directives.

C. The patient's wishes in regard to refusing or executing an advanced directive will be documented in the medical record.

FIGURE 7–6 Patient Self-Determination Act of 1990 (PSDA)

PROXY DECISION-MAKING STANDARDS

The courts have not made their decisions on the basis of personhood criteria but rather have created standards for the allowance of decisions by proxy. When an individual is not competent to refuse treatment, often the physician, hospital, or a family member may seek resolution of the problem from the courts prior to implementing a decision. Under the doctrine of **parens patriae,** the state accepts these cases on the basis of a legitimate duty, abiding in the principles of beneficence and nonmaleficence. This duty requires the protection of citizens under legal disability from harms they cannot themselves avoid. In cases where individuals were incompetent to decide for themselves, the courts have generally used one of two proxy decision-making standards, that of best interest, and substituted judgment.

The **best-interest standard** most often takes into account such tangible factors as harms and benefits, physical and fiscal risks. In health care, the courts might rely on such truisms as "Health is better than illness," and "Life is preferable to death." In cases where children have been denied life-preserving care by their parents, the state has often overturned the parental decisions based on the best-interest standard.

The **substituted-judgment standard,** unlike the best-interest standard, maintains that the decision about treatment or nontreatment must remain that of the patient, based on the principle of autonomy. The fact that a patient is incompetent to make a decision for himself does not take from him the right to self-determination. A substitute is selected who is required to act in proxy for the patient—that is, to make the decision that the incompetent patient would have made if the patient had been competent. In the case of Karen Ann, her father could draw upon the experiences of her previous life to determine her wants in this particular case. If patients, while competent, have clearly expressed their will through conversations or advanced directives as to their disposition in these cases, the substituted-judgment seems a rational approach.

Complicating these issues are two groups of cases, one involving competent individuals who become incompetent without expressing their wishes, and a second group, the mentally retarded who may never have met the criterion of competence. What standard best serves these patients?

These two groups seem best served by the **standard of best interest,** where the court bases its decision on the principles of beneficence and nonmaleficence rather than on patient autonomy. This appears to provide a sounder basis for decision making, especially if the individual has never been in a position to have made an autonomous decision.

The Joseph Saikewicz case is an example of the standard of best interest as it is used for patients who are incompetent to make decisions in regard to acceptance or refusal of treatment.[20] Joseph, who was profoundly retarded and had the intellectual capacity of a three-year-old, had lived his 67 years of life in a mental institution. In 1976, he was diagnosed as having a terminal form of leukemia. Even with aggressive chemotherapy, his chances for a remission would be only 30 percent, and the remission would only extend his life for a short period of perhaps another year. Without the chemotherapy he was expected to live for several months before succumbing to infection.

The problem with providing the chemotherapy for Joseph was that the treatment required potent drugs, which caused nausea and discomfort. Moreover, because the staff could not make the patient understand the nature of his illness or the reason for the treatment, he would probably need to be physically restrained. The institution where Joseph was treated appealed to the courts for guidance in the case. Two physicians were called to testify and spoke against the administration of the chemotherapy. The court ruled that the chemotherapy not be given, and the decision was appealed to the State Supreme Court, which concurred with the lower court ruling. Joseph Saikewicz had died from pneumonia prior to the time the higher court had issued it's full opinion. The court ruled that a guardian could be assigned to make the judgment, but that the judgment be based on the best interest of the patient. To assure that the patient's interests were considered, the court required that an adversarial judicial hearing be held as opposed to reliance on doctors, families, and hospital committees—as proposed in the Quinlan case.

INFORMED NONCONSENT

In the cases of Karen Ann Quinlan, Nancy Cruzan, and Joseph Saikewicz, the patients were considered incompetent to make their own decisions and needed others to determine whether treatment should be continued or withdrawn. Recently, there have been a series of cases involving competent patients who understood the nature of their conditions and the consequences of refusing care and have chosen informed nonconsent.

William Bartling was a 75-year-old chronic pulmonary disease patient with four other terminal illnesses. There was no question as to his competence when he requested to be removed from his ventilator. The hospital refused his request due to the fact that if the device was removed it would surely hasten his death. When the hospital refused to accept his living will as a rationale for removing the ventilator, he appealed to the courts, who affirmed the institutional decision. On several occasions Bartling attempted to remove the ventilator himself until he was placed in restraints. Although both Bartling and his wife made repeated requests in regard to his desire to refuse the care, he spent the last six months of his life on the ventilator and died before the appeals court overturned the lower court decision and ruled in his favor.[21]

Elizabeth Bouvia was a 28-year-old quadriplegic suffering from severe cerebral palsy. During her hospitalizations, she asked that her pain be controlled and that she be allowed to starve herself to death. Physicians and hospital authorities refused her request, and she was force-fed through a nasogastric tube to maintain body weight. She requested that the feeding be stopped, and the hospital refused even though her competency was not questioned. Bouvia went to court several times during the next several years, making media headlines and becoming a symbol of the **right-to-die movement.** The lower courts affirmed the hospital decisions, but these decisions were finally overturned by the appeals court. The court in its ruling determined that the fact that Ms. Bouvia was young and therefore had a potential for a long life was essentially irrelevant. The decision stated that the time allotted for continued life was not the issue, only the perceived quality of that life, and that "If a right exists, it matters not what motivates its exercise." Although the Bouvia case did not affirm a basic right to die, it did become a landmark decision regarding the right to informed nonconsent.[22]

These cases seem to indicate a growing consensus in regard to the allowance of personal autonomy and informed nonconsent. The legal rights of patients to refuse medical treatment have been upheld in over 80 court decisions.[23] The courts appear to be moving closer to the view that patients are entitled to be allowed to die. Several critical elements were reinforced by the court decisions:

1. The acuity of the patient is irrelevant to the allowance of treatment refusal. The patient's right to refuse care is not dependent upon having a terminal illness.

2. The patient's own perceived view of his/her quality of life and the treatment requirements necessary to preserve it are of paramount importance. The fact that Elizabeth Bouvia could potentially live for another four decades and be a productive citizen could not overcome her autonomous choice to refuse care.

3. There is no meaningful legal distinction between mechanical life support and nasogastric feeding; both are invasive.

4. Distinctions between withholding and withdrawing care are legally irrelevant.

DNR ORDERS (Do Not Resuscitate)

Cardiopulmonary Resuscitation (CPR) and advanced cardiac life support (ACLS) are interventions that could theoretically be offered to all patients within the hospital. By the 1970s, it became obvious that it was not in the best interest of certain patient groups to be resuscitated, and hospitals began to initiate policies governing **DNR (Do Not Resuscitate) Orders.** Due to uncertainty as to appropriate criteria for selecting these patients, the late 70s and 80s were a period of confusion in which health care support staff were left to find their way through an ambiguous maze of verbal orders as well as orders for slow codes, partial codes, purple dots, etc. Figure 7–7, differentiates between these various types of DNR orders. DNR policies are now required of all hospitals by the Joint Commission for the Accreditation of

Code: A call for cardiopulmonary resuscitation efforts. In the hospital setting, a code would usually contain all the elements of advanced cardiac life support which includes, oxygenation, ventilation, cardiac massage, electroshock as necessary, and emergency drugs. These are sometimes announced as "Code Blue" or some other designation to signal the emergency team of the need to respond.

No Code: DNR (Do Not Resuscitate) A written order placed in the medical chart to avoid the use of cardiopulmonary resuscitation efforts. In previous times, often the charts were labled with devices such as "Red Tags," or "Purple Dots" to designate DNR status.

Slow Codes: This is a practice whereby the health care team slows down the process of emergency resuscitation so as to appear to be providing the care but in actual fact is only providing an illusion. The intent of the practice is more for family comfort than patient benefit.

Chemical Code: Similar in intent to the slow code. In this practice, the team provides the drugs needed for resuscitation but does not provide the other services. There is a real question as to whether slow codes, chemical codes, other forms of resuscitation that contain only partial efforts are appropriate for anything other than theatrics.

FIGURE 7–7 Language of DNR

1. DNR orders should be documented in the written medical record.

2. DNR orders should specify the exact nature of the treatments to be withheld.

3. Patients, when they are able, should participate in DNR decisions. Their involvement and wishes should be documented in the medical record.

4. Decisions to withhold CPR should be discussed with the health care team.

5. DNR status should be reviewed on a regular basis.

FIGURE 7–8 DNR Guidelines

Health Care Organizations. Figure 7–8 provides general guidelines that one might expect for the establishment of DNR policies within a modern health care facility.

Even given the wide use and acceptance of DNR orders, the selection of patients still raises some concern. In our age of cost containment and stretched resources, do DNR patients belong in intensive care units? Studies show that these patients in ICU are sicker, have longer stays, have poorer prognosis, consume more resources (both human and fiscal), and have a higher mortality rate than do non-DNR patients. Thirty-nine percent of the ICU patient deaths occur with those who have DNR orders.[24]

In their *Guidelines on the Termination of Life-Sustaining Treatment and the Care of the Dying,* the Hastings Center authors concluded that the intent of DNR orders did not preclude either the use of any other treatment modalities or admission and treatment in an intensive care unit. When treatment (either curative or palliative) cannot be obtained in other units outside intensive care, the patient's rights to autonomy, beneficence, and nonmaleficence, coupled with the requirements of fidelity, make the ICU usage a reasonable choice.[25]

The initiation of DNR orders is best performed after an understanding by physicians, patients, family, and staff has been reached. This is an area in which value preference will make a great deal of difference. In one case where the physician was attempting to broach the subject of placing a DNR order, he began by telling the patient that if he had another event, the chances of CPR being effective would be one in a thousand. The patient replied by asking a question in regard to his chances if CPR were not initiated. This patient wanted whatever chances there might be and wasn't interested in statistics.[26] Although patient/provider discussion in regard to DNR orders would, in theory, facilitate autonomous control by the patient, research has consistently shown that only about 20 percent of the patients with DNR orders discussed their resuscitative preference prior to the order being implemented.

BABY DOE

Unlike the informed nonconsent of autonomous adults or the substituted-judgment cases involving those who are irreversibly incompetent to make decisions are those situations involving withholding or withdrawing care from infants. No decisions are more filled with anguish for all involved, parents and health care providers alike. In the Spring of 1982, an infant known as Baby Doe was born with an esophageal-tracheal fistula and trisomy 21, a form of mental retardation known commonly as Down syndrome. The esophageal-tracheal fistula needed immediate surgery if the infant was to be fed. The decision of whether to do the surgery would not have been questioned for a "normal infant." The physicians split in their recommendations as to whether to provide the surgery in this case, the parents with court concurrence elected to refuse the surgery on behalf of their child, and the infant died. The parents based their decision on their view that it would not be in their son's best interest to survive, since he would always be severely retarded.[27]

In March 1983, in response to this case and others like it, the United States Department of Health and Human Services issued an "Interim Final Rule," which directed that all health care facilities dealing with infants less than one year of age and who received federal funding prominently display an antidiscrimination notice protecting these infants. The notice provided a "handicapped infant hotline" for those who might witness cases where infants were receiving less than *customary medical care.*"[28] Anyone in the nursery could then call and complain about care, and the federal government would send representatives to investigate the allegations. The fear of "Baby Doe squads" descending upon the health care facility and involving themselves in what had previously been a rather private parent/physician arena of decision making had a serious chilling effect upon deliberations having to do with infant care. The force of the notices was to place a potential conflict between the law and the moral obligations of the health care providers. Legal duties in and of themselves do not establish moral duties and visa versa.

The definition of "customary medical care" is sufficiently vague as to imply the necessity to preserve life regardless of the potential quality or value of that life to the individual. It appeared that medicine was to be forced away from any decision-making role in regard to these issues, even in those instances where infants were born with complete absence of vital parts of their brains. The national media picked up the Baby Doe issue and began to relate it to the civil rights movement and the holocaust. This feeling that something was basically wrong and that the government had a duty to protect these infants was forcefully stated by the conservative columnist Patrick Buchanan in the following interesting, although overblown, "slippery slope" argument or "wedge" line of reasoning.

> Once, however, we embrace this utilitarian ethic—that man has the sovereign right to decide who is entitled to life and who is not—we have boarded a passenger train on which there are no scheduled stops between here and Birkenau.
>
> Once we accept that there are certain classes, i.e., unwanted, unborn children, unwanted infants who are retarded or handicapped, etc., whose lives are unworthy of legal protection, upon what moral high ground do we stand to decry when Dr. Himmler slaps us on the back, and asks us if he can include Gypsies and Jews?[29]

As with most important issues, responsible forces lined up on both sides. Opposing the regulations were groups such as the American Academy of Pediatrics and the American Medical Association. In support were groups such as the American Association of Retarded Citizens, who felt that the decision to provide care should be neutral in respect to handicap. In other words, if a "normal infant" would have received the surgery, then infants with handicaps should also. Of the almost four million infants born each year, approximately 10 percent are born prematurely or with major birth defects. Modern surgery and neonatal care has been rather miraculous; however many of these infants still face life severely handicapped. In the investigations of more than 1,500 hotline reports following the Baby Doe case, the government found only three cases in which infants were allegedly being denied appropriate care.

In 1984, Congress passed the Child Abuse Amendment, which provided guidelines in regard to when it was appropriate to withhold medically indicated treatment from these infants. The physician is not obliged to provide care beyond that of a palliative nature when, in the treating physician's reasonable medical judgment, any of the following circumstances apply.

1. The infant is chronically and irreversibly comatose.
2. The provision of such treatment would merely
    a. prolong dying.
    b. not be effective in ameliorating or correcting ALL of the infant's life-threatening conditions.
    c. be futile in terms of survival.
3. The provision of such treatment would be virtually futile in terms of the survival of the infant and the treatment itself under such circumstances would be inhumane.[30]

In 1986, following the recommendations of the President's Commission on Medical Ethics, the Supreme Court of the United States ruled that the Baby Doe regulations were not authorized under Section 504 of the Rehabilitation Act of 1973. The court emphasized that child protection was a state responsibility and that the primary decision makers for their children should be parents, provided that these decisions were in the children's best interest. With this ruling, the federal government was out of the Baby Doe business, and parents and physicians once again could wrestle with these problems somewhat out of the public eye.

Regardless of who the primary decision makers are, the ethical problems remain. Whereas parents have a right to privacy, and to be left alone in their decisions in regard to their children, this is not an absolute right and does not extend to child abuse. What is the child's best interest in these cases?

If the infant's mental and physical handicaps are overwhelming, it would be inhumane to provide life-extending care and to salvage the infant to a life whose only awareness is that of pain and suffering. On the other hand, to refuse care to a child on the whimsy of being dissatisfied with a particular model is equally distasteful. The right choice for these babies is easy to determine at the extremes, but it becomes a true problem when deciding for the infants—where it is not clear—as to what constitutes their best interest. Perhaps these are cases that are best served by basing the judgments upon the for **quality of life issue,** or personhood. In order to have value, life must contain some aspects of quality, such as awareness, and the potential for human relationships. This view is in keeping with the writings of Richard McCormick, a Jesuit priest who defends a quality-of-life determination.

> It is neither inhuman nor un-Christian to say that there comes a point where an individual's condition itself represents the negation of any truly human—i.e., relational—potential. When that point is reached, is not the best treatment no treatment?[31]

Translated into the language of personhood, an infant who has no present or future potential for self-awareness or relationships can be said to have no interests at all. It then becomes incomprehensible to provide life-extending care based on the child's best interests, as it makes no difference to the child whether the equipment is maintained for five minutes or five years.

SUMMARY

Medical science can now save biological life so effectively that we have been forced away from using a cardiopulmonary definition of death to the certification of death by brain function. We have also as a product of our technology and therapeutics moved into a time of being able to fend off brain death, only to expose the patient to continued misery and suffering. Health care providers have reached a quandary in which the duty to respect and preserve life comes into direct conflict with the duty to prevent and relieve pain.

In this chapter we have examined several classes of patients for whom decisions of withdrawing and withholding care have been reasoned through. These decisions have gained some cultural, legal, and ethical acceptance. Reasoning for the profoundly handicapped infant, the PVS patient, those who chose informed nonconsent, and the mentally retarded each require a different basis. In some areas such as the abortion controversy, no consensus exists within our society. In some instances, the framework of what is to be done has been postponed and the issue has become, instead, who is to decide.

Some instances of nontreatment seem to have gained acceptance and are rather noncontroversial. The 98-year-old with severe dementia and not a relative in the world who contracts pneumonia might be allowed to die quietly. The real questions in regard to health provider duty do not lie in the extremes, such as an infant born with no brain inside it's skull, but in the middle ground where there will be a potential for personhood and meaningful life. In the extreme cases where no potential exists, or where the best interests of the individual seem best served by withholding or withdrawing treatment, a form of passive euthanasia has been allowed. **Euthanasia,** which literally means a gentle or easy death, has been divided into two major groupings, passive and active. This chapter has been involved in the issues of passive euthanasia, the process of doing nothing to prolong life or fend off death. Active euthanasia, as defined by the active participation of ending life, is currently forbidden by the laws of all 50 states, as well as most codes of ethical conduct. Active euthanasia will form the basis of the discussion found in Chapter 8.

CLARIFICATION EXERCISES:

A. The case involves a young, ventilator-dependent quadriplegic patient who, after being shunted about to various facilities, sought to have his ventilator unhooked. The court recognized him as a competent adult and allowed the withdrawal of his life support.

In this particular case, neither the court, the health care providers, the right-to-life movement, nor the churches came forward to argue that the ventilator should be continued. After he had gained permission to withdraw from life support, the patient decided against the action and still remains on the ventilator.

The question that this case brings forward is whether the young man's demand to have the "right to die" was real or just another way of saying "Do you care about me?" A secondary question that is equally problematic is whether the acceptance of his request was based on a respect for his personal autonomy, or was it just an answer to the "Do you care about me?" question with a "no!"

Respond to the idea that our current acceptance of "a right to die," especially for those who are unconscious and need a proxy decision maker, is a rather slippery slope that may in the future be used not to protect individual autonomy or privacy but rather as a facade to rid us of individuals whose lives we do not value.

B. Differentiate between the various lines of reasoning and arguments needed to decide the following types of cases in regard to withdrawing or withholding care:

1. Persistent Vegetative State cases
2. Profoundly Retarded Patient cases
3. Baby Doe cases
4. Informed nonconsent cases

Which of the above case types is best served by proxy judgments, and if so, what form—"best interest" or "substituted judgment"?

C. In 1972, the philosopher Joseph Fletcher issued a paper listing the characteristics of a person. The following are taken from his positive criteria:

1. Minimal IQ: Mere biological life, before minimal intelligence is achieved or after it is irreversibly lost, is without person status.
2. Self-Awareness: the development of self-awareness in babies is what we watch and take such joy in. In psychotherapy, the lack of self-awareness would represent grave pathology.
3. Self Control: An individual not only not controllable by others (without restraint), but also not in his or her own control.
4. A sense of time: memories, a feeling of now, and expectations for the future.
5. The capability to Relate to Others: Interpersonal relationships seem essential to being a person in any meaningful sense.
6. Concern for Others: Extra-ego orientation is a vital characteristic of a "real person."
7. Curiosity: A person is a learner; total indifference is inhuman.
8. Communication: Utter alienation or disconnection from others is not a characteristic of humanity.
9. Neo-cortical Function: Personal reality is dependent upon cerebral function; it forms the basis between life in a biographical and biological sense.
10. Idiosyncrasy: Humans are distinct; to be a person is to have identity, to be recognizable or callable by name.

Rank order the list from most important to least important in your view of what makes up a person. Check those that you would consider to be essential in regard to personhood. If you feel that a particular characteristic is essential, you must be willing to deny those who do not possess it the rights and privileges of person status.

In regard to the personhood criteria that you have selected, state how this would affect your decisions in the following cases.

Nancy Cruzan

Joseph Saikewicz

Elizabeth Bouvia

Baby Doe

In regard to KoKo the Gorilla, who uses sign language to communicate with humans and appears to have a kitten that she cares about and misses when it is gone, what is her level of personhood?

If an angel or alien appeared out of the sky and had all the elements, that you said were essential to being a person, would the alien have all the rights and privileges of a person?

D. Assuming that Baby Doe would have grown up to know himself, know those around him, walk, talk and play, and perhaps even go to school, was the decision not to provide the surgery ethical? Regardless of how you answer, justify your decision using ethical criteria. Also note that legal decisions are ethics neutral, and visa versa: Something truly can be legally correct, medically correct, socially correct, and morally reprehensible. Ask Dr. Mengele (Nazi war criminal who performed ghoulish experiments in the death camps), for he surely felt that relative to his society what he was doing was socially, medically, and legally correct.

E. Mr. Joseph was a 75-year-old chronic obstructive disease patient. He was in the hospital because of an upper respiratory tract infection. He and his wife had requested that CPR not be performed should he require it. A DNR order was written in the charts. In his room on the third floor he was being maintained with antibiotics, fluids, and oxygen and seemed to be doing better. However, Mr. Joseph's oxygen was inadvertently turned up, and this caused him to go into respiratory failure. When found by the therapist, he was in terrible distress and lay gasping in his bed.

Should Mr. Joseph be transferred to intensive care, where his respiratory failure can be treated by a ventilator and his oxygen level can be monitored? Whatever your answer, provide an ethical rationale.

F. In a recent nursing journal question-and-answer column the individual asked the question as to what his duty was when a physician wrote DNR orders for all her AIDS patients, even though it was known that the patients wanted everything done that was possible. When questioned, the physician just shrugged and said "*I know what is best for my patients.*"

How would you advise the nurse?

G. In a recent case, an 86-year-old female was being maintained by a ventilator. The physicians concluded that the treatment was futile, that it would not reverse the underlying disease process or restore the woman to a state of acceptable function. They approached the husband in regard to removing the ventilator. He informed them that his wife would have wanted to be kept alive even in a persistent vegetative state. What should the health care providers do?

REFERENCES AND SUGGESTED READING

1. Albert Schweitzer, as quoted in *Doctor's Dilemmas: Medical Ethics and Contempory Science* (Great Britain: Harvester Press Limited, 1985), 22.
2. Morris Cohen, *The Faith of a Liberal* (New York: Henry Holt and Company, 1946), 287.
3. Ruth Macklin, *Mortal Choices* (Boston: Houghton Mifflin Company, 1987), 7–8.

4. Nancy Cruzan gravestone.
5. Ad Hoc Committee of the Harvard Medical School to Examine the Definition of Death, "A Definition of Irreversible Coma," *Journal of the American Medical Association* 246, no. 19 (Nov. 13, 1981).
6. Thomas Furlow, "Tyranny of Technology; A Physician looks at Euthanasia," *The Humanist* 34, 4 (1974): 6–8.
7. John Sorenson, *Determination of Death: The Need for a Higher Brain Concept in Medical Ethics,* ed. Monagle and Thomasma (Rockville, MD:, Aspen Publishers, 1988).
8. *In Re Quinlan,* 70 New Jersey 10, 355 A2d 647, 79 ALR 3d 205 (1976).
9. 1957 Encyclical "Prolongation of Life" as quoted in Brody Howard, *Ethical Decisions in Modern Medicine* (Boston: Little, Brown and Company, 1981), 91.
10. Gerald Kelly, *Medico-moral Problems* (St. Louis: Catholic Hospital Association, 1957), 129.
11. G. Meilaender, "On Removing Food and Water: Against the Stream," *Hastings Center Report* 14 (1984) 11–13.
12. Joseph Fletcher, "Indicators of Personhood," *Hastings Center Report* (1972): 1–4.
13. Joel Feinberg, "The Problem of Personhood," in T. Beauchamp, and L. Walters, *Contemporary Issues In Bioethics* (Belmont, CA: Wadsworth Publishing Co. 1982), 108–115.
14. Nancy's Father's statement.
15. *Cruzan v. Director, Missouri Department of Health,* 110 US SCt, 2841 (1990).
16. Agile Freedman, "Right-to-Die Guidelines Murky in Most States," *Health Week Briefing Paper,* Phillips Medical Systems (March 1990): 30–33
17. Society for the Right to Die, *Handbook of Living Will Laws* (New York: Society for the Right to Die, 1987).
18. Anne Allen, "Advanced Directives Provide Answers for Tough Questions," *Journal of Post Anesthesia Nursing,* 7, no 3 (June 1992): 183–185.
19. George Annas, "Transferring the Ethical Hot Potato," *Hastings Center Report* (November 1987), 20–23.
20. *Superintendent of Belchertown State School v. Saikewicz,* 373 Mass 728, 370 NE2d 417 (1977).
21. *Bartling v. Superior Court,* 163 Cal. App3d 186, 195 (1984).
22. *Bouvia v. Superior Court,* 179 Cal. App3d 1127 (1986).
23. Thomas Scully and Celia Scully, *Playing God* (New York: Simon and Schuster, 1987), 92–123.
24. Barbara Edwards, "Does the DNR Patient Belong in the ICU?" in *Critical Nursing Clinics of North America.* W. B. Saunders (September 1990): 473–479.
25. Council on Ethical and Judicial Affairs, "Guidelines for the Appropriate Use of Do-Not-Resuscitate Orders," *Journal of the American Medical Association* 265, no. 14 (April 10, 1991): 1868–1871.
26. Thomas Scully and Celia Scully, *Playing God* (New York: Simon and Schuster, 1987), 23.
27. Mary Rhoden, "Treating Baby Doe: The Ethics of Uncertainty," *Hastings Center Report* (August 1986): 34–42.
28. J.C. Moscop and R.L. Saldanha, "The Baby Doe Rule: Still a Threat," *Hastings Center Report* (April 1986): 8–12.
29. Patrick Buchanan, "The Dividing Line," an editorial in the *New York Times,* 15 November 1983.
30. Ruth Macklin, *Mortal Choices: Ethical Dilemmas in Modern Medicine* (Boston: Houghton Mifflin Company, 1987), 123.
31. Richard McCormick, "To Save or Let Die: The Dilemma of Modern Medicine," *Journal of the American Medical Association* 229 (1979): 172–76.

CHAPTER 8

Euthanasia: Practice and Principles

Instructional Goal

The major instructional goal for this chapter is to gain an understanding of the national debate in regard to euthanasia. The chapter will differentiate between the variety of forms that this practice takes and look at the various arguments for and against the adoption of the practice in modern health care.

Instructional Objectives

At the end of this chapter the reader should understand and be able to:

1. Define and differentiate between active and passive euthanasia.
2. Discuss the two major arguments for the adoption of a "right to die."
3. Discuss the religious and nonreligious arguments against the adoption of active euthanasia as a practice of modern health care.
4. Outline the current position taken by the health care community in regard to the practice of both active and passive euthanasia.
5. Outline the nature of the Hospice Movement in the United States and discuss how this may impact on the debate regarding euthanasia.
6. Discuss the current ambiguity between the law and court decisions regarding mercy killing in the United States.

Glossary

Active Euthanasia: Actively assisting the process of death.

Euthanasia: Easy death; death without suffering; painlessly induced death.

Hospice Movement: The development of centers for providing palliative care for the terminally ill that focus on the process of relieving pain and suffering.

Involuntary Euthanasia: Actively assisting the process of death for someone who has not requested assistance.

112

Medicide: The termination of life by a medical specialist.

Mercy Killing: Active voluntary euthanasia.

Palliative Care: Care that is designed not to cure but to provide relief from pain and suffering.

Passive Euthanasia Ceasing therapies that prolong life so that death can occur.

Sophistry: A plausible but misleading or fallacious argument; subtle rhetoric designed to mislead.

Voluntary Euthanasia: Actively assisting the process of death for someone who has requested assistance in the dying process.

LEGAL AND SOCIAL STANDING OF EUTHANASIA

Do not go gentle into that good night,
Old age should burn and rave at close of day;
Rage, rage against the dying of the light.

Dylan Thomas

The Moment had come. With a nod from Janet I turned on the ECG and said, "Now" Janet hit the Mercitron's switch with the outer edge of her palm. In about ten seconds her eyelids began to flicker and droop. She looked at me and said, "Thank you, thank you." I replied at once as her eyelids closed, "Have a nice trip."[1]

Jack Kevorkian, M.D.

In June of 1990, Janet Adkins ended her life with the help of Dr. Jack Kevorkian. She killed herself in a van parked in a secluded park using a suicide machine (Mercitron) created by the doctor. With her death, the controversy of **active euthanasia** once again came to the fore in national debate. The right to choose death has become an important issue. In our rapidly aging society there is a great underlying fear of being old, abandoned, and facing a lingering death filled with pain or unawareness. High-profile cases such as Karen Ann Quinlan and Nancy Cruzan have made the public question the wisdom of prolonging lives that appear to have no value to the individual. Dr. Kevorkian himself invisions a whole new specialty to be known as **Medicide**[2]. He argues that assisted suicide with the support and direction of a medical specialist might be a merciful option for the following categories of suicide:[3]

Obligatory Assisted Suicide: A category that includes individuals who must be put to death. Examples might be inmates on death row.

Obligatory Suicide: These would be individuals who are irrevocably condemned to kill themselves. An example might be followers of the Jim Jones religious cult of Guyana.

Optional Suicide: This would be a category of individuals who are in no way ill but who have arbitrarily and irrevocably decided upon death.

Optional Assisted Suicide: The individual would not be ill but would be facing a situation in which death was preferable to living. A historical example might be the Zealots of Masada.

Suicide by Proxy: This category would be for those who are incapable of giving informed consent. The decision would be that of another. Fetuses, infants, and minor children would fall into this class.

Although Kevorkian, his death machine, and attendant legal problems currently assume center stage in the controversy, euthanasia is by no means a recent issue in the United States. Figure 8–1 outlines the criteria for legalization of euthanasia found in a bill brought before the New York State General Assembly and defeated in 1947. Similar bills are being prepared in several jurisdictions across the country today.[4]

The ethical and legal issues of withholding or withdrawing life support have been reasonably worked out in cases such as those of Karen Ann Quinlan and Nancy Cruzan, and there appears to be some consensus for allowing health care providers to participate under these circumstances in **passive euthanasia.** The allowance of a deadly process to proceed without intervention is generally acceptable in the United States when the treatment is futile, and no possibility of patient benefit exists. Every day, in a hundred hospital settings, "DNR" orders are written in charts, respirators are disconnected, IV lines are removed, and proposed surgeries are canceled. Over half the states today have legislation covering advanced directives, and many specifically provide that a patient or proxy can authorize the withholding or withdrawal of life-support systems. Although still somewhat controversial, the issue today does not revolve around passive euthanasia, or the standing aside and allowing the terminal patient to die. Figure 8–2 is "The Old Man's Prayer," written by Bob Richards, which elegantly states the socially agreed upon case for passive euthanasia.[5]

1. Any sane person over twenty years old, suffering from an incurably painful and fatal disease, may petition a court of record for euthanasia, in a signed and attested document with an affidavit from the attending physician that in his opinion the disease is incurable;

2. The court may appoint a commission of three, of whom at least two shall be physicians, to investigate all aspects of the case and to report back to the courts whether the patient understands the purpose of his petition and comes under the provisions of the act;

3. Upon a favorable report by the commission the court shall grant the petition, and, if it is still wanted by the patient, euthanasia may be adminsitered by a physician or any other person chosen by the patient or by the commission. (4)

FIGURE 8–1 Euthanasia Bill: New York, 1947

OLD MAN'S PRAYER

Pardon me, doctor, but may I die?
I know your oath requires you try
As long as there's a spark of life
To keep it there with tube and knife;

To do cut-downs and heart massages,
Tracheotomies and gavages.
But here I am, well past four-score.
I've lived my lifetime (and a little more)

I've raised my children, buried my wife.
My friends are gone, so spare the knife.
This is the way it seems to me
I deserve a little dignity . . .

Of slipping gently off to sleep
And no one has the right to keep
Me from my God: when the call's this clear
No mortal man should keep me here.

Your motive's noble, but now I pray
You'll read my eyes, what my lips can't say
Listen to my heart! You'll hear it cry;
"Pardon me, Doctor, but may I die?" (5)

FIGURE 8–2

However, our system currently holds that there is an important distinction between assisting the death of patients and letting them die, even though the outcome seems the same. The American Medical Association Code of Ethics states that, except in special circumstances, it is illegal to deliberately cause the death of another person. The AMA does not, however, have the same admonition (special circumstances) against allowing a person to die. In the one case, you are initiating the process that brings about the death, in the other, you are just allowing a deadly process, which you did not initiate, to continue. The one case is viewed as morally wrong and the other as morally permissible. Critics of this view feel the difference is a matter of **sophistry,** for inherent in the decision to do nothing is the decision for death. Is the removal of the ventilator, and IV lines, and feeding tubes from a patient who cannot breathe, or eat for himself any less a complicity in the resulting death, than if you provided a bolus of morphine to hasten the process? If there is no difference, is the bolus the more humane act?

The term **euthanasia** comes from the Greek for *good death* and in English has taken the meaning of easy death or the *painless inducement of quick death.* The concept of easy death is further divided into two categories: passive euthanasia, which involves doing nothing to preserve life, and active euthanasia, which requires actions that speed the process of dying. Euthanasia is further divided, depending upon whether the process is initiated by patient request, and is therefore voluntary or involuntarily implemented without patient permission.

Involuntary euthanasia, which ignores the individual's autonomous rights and could potentially bring about the death of an unwilling victim, is not easily distinguished from murder. There is very little disagreement in our society that involuntary euthanasia is morally indefensible. The focus of the current controversy that rages through our health care system is whether there is a moral difference between active and passive **voluntary euthanasia.** Several states have put statutes before the citizens in regard to legalizing voluntary active euthanasia, but thus far none have succeeded.

It is perhaps important to differentiate between killing (involuntary euthanasia) and suicide, although neither provides the focus of this chapter, which is centered on the question of allowing voluntary active euthanasia. Tom Beauchamp offers a precise definition of suicide that separates it from the process of passive or active voluntary euthanasia. A person has committed suicide when:

1. That person brings about his or her own death;

2. Others do not coerce him or her to do the action; and

3. Death is caused by conditions arranged by the person for the purpose of bringing about his or her death.[6]

Although the frequency of occurrence is unknown, it is not a rare event for physicians to prescribe sleeping and pain medications for hopelessly ill patients who request them, knowing full well that their intended use is suicide. Some physicians see this as the last act in a continuum of care. As noted above, suicide differs from euthanasia in that the health care provider does not participate in the act of bringing about death. Any physician who becomes involved in the suicide of a patient must first be assured that the patient is indeed in a hopeless situation and not just suffering from treatable depression, common in individuals with terminal illnesses.

One of the real problems with Dr. Kevorkian and his death machine (the Mercitron) is determining whether his patients are committing suicide, whether he is practicing voluntary euthanasia, or is he perhaps murdering these unfortunates. When he builds his machines, advertises in newspapers, (see Fig. 8–3), videotapes the events, purchases the lethal dosages, arranges for undisturbed sites, puts in IV lines, and finally arranges for postmortem press conferences, has he stepped beyond being a mere observer when the patients push the button to release the drugs?

Some would find the acts of Dr. Kevorkian similar to the political terrorist who bombs buildings and buses in order to bring about political change. These seeming criminal acts have at times brought about positive political change. Kevorkian may be the harbinger of change and usher in a new specialty known as obiatry, practitioners of which would legally perform euthanasia in our society. Perhaps in the future there will be obiatry clinics in every major city. However, just as some terrorist acts usher in positive developments, others do nothing more than murder innocents and leave no permanent positive effects for their efforts. In a recent news article, the ethicist Arthur Caplan argues that Kevorkian's campaign of mercy takes its heaviest toll on the poor, the disabled and women and that his clients are more victims than beneficiaries.[8] Perhaps Kevorkian is nothing more than a serial killer

Is someone in your family
terminally ill?

Does he or she wish to die —
and with dignity?

CALL PHYSICIAN CONSULTANT

(Telephone number)[7]

FIGURE 8–3 Kevorkian Classified Newspaper Ad

with a gimmick. History has yet to determine whether Kevorkian is in the forefront of change or is just a wild, uncontrolled eccentric who captures headlines and eventually fades from the attention of the media.

A health care practitioner who deliberately hastens the death of a patient under the guise of "mercy killing" has entered into a practice prohibited under the homicide laws. Common and criminal law regard life as sacred and inalienable and look at any premeditated killing as homicide. "Consent and humanitarian motive" is never a defense under the law for murder. "He nonetheless acts with malice if he is able to comprehend that society prohibits his act regardless of his personal beliefs."[9]

In the early 1980s, Holland became the first modern nation to tolerate active health care provider involvement in the deaths of patients. During the 1980's the practice was illegal but allowed, and it has now received legal sanction. The Dutch have prescribed a series of specific conditions that must be met prior to assisting the death of a patient: First, the consent must be free, conscious, explicit, and persistent. Second, the physician and patient must both agree that the suffering is intolerable, and that other measures for relief have all been exhausted. Third, a second physician must be in agreement, and all relevant facts in the case must be recorded. If the individual is a child, the parental consent must be obtained.[10]

While illegal in all jurisdictions of the United States, recent polls show that 64 percent of those questioned favor physician-assisted suicide. In other studies it was found that, even among religious groups with strong admonitions against suicide, there is a majority sentiment in favor of physician-assisted deliverance. This public support for euthanasia, even in the face of illegality, is in evidence in several cases where family members have assisted in the death of individuals in chronic pain.[11]

MERCY KILLING

An elderly woman with Alzheimer's disease that had progressed to the point that she could no longer do simple chores and whose vocabulary had shrunk to two words (fire and pain), which she screamed in German, was shot by her husband of 33 years. Hans Florian claimed that he shot his wife because he was 17 years her senior and he feared that he might die first and leave her alone.[12] Under American law, he had no legal right to harm his wife and could have been brought up on the charge of murder. After considering the issues involved, the Florida Grand Jury refused to indict him.

In Michigan, 73-year-old Bertram Harper was acquitted of murdering his terminally ill wife even though he admitted placing a plastic bag over her head. He and his wife had checked into a motel with the intention of her committing suicide. When her efforts failed, he placed a plastic bag over her head to smother her.[13]

In both the Florian and Harper cases the facts were clear that, indeed, the men had participated in ending their wives' lives, yet in both cases they were not held accountable for the actions. What these cases indicate is a reservoir of public sentiment for **mercy killing** under certain circumstances. The practice of mercy killing is on the rise in the United States, with more cases being reported between 1980 and 1990 than in the previous half century. What is most interesting is that, in almost all instances, the defendants have not been imprisoned for the offense. Instead the courts have found the individuals not guilty on the grounds of temporary insanity or have mandated long periods of probation.

Although the law is rather unequivocal in regard to the practice of active euthanasia, the court decisions have been quite ambiguous. This may be a proper stance for the law in that its adamant negative position provides a deterrent to all considerations of the practice, and forces deliberation of the merits on a case-by-case basis. But under what circumstances is euthanasia justifiable? Is it permissible to kill the terminally ill? How about those who are not terminally ill but only have lost their appetite for life? Even if society decides that citizens have a right not only to life, liberty and property, but also to death, what part do health care practitioners play in this right? Would the role of public euthanizer have a chilling effect upon the healing arts?

One highly publicized account of practitioner mercy killing known as "It's Over, Debbie," involved a gynecology resident rotating through a large private hospital. The physician was awakened by the nurse on duty and told that a patient dying of ovarian cancer was having difficulty getting rest. When the physician entered the patient's room, he found her sitting in bed, emaciated and in severe air hunger. The patient's only words to the physician were "Let's get this over with." The physician left the room and instructed the nurse to draw up 20 milligrams of morphine sulfate into a syringe, which he then injected intravenously into the patient after telling her and a woman visitor that "it would let her rest," and "to say good-bye." The woman died of respiratory failure within a few minutes.[14]

In that the reporting of this incident was in a "letters" format to a medical journal, there is some doubt that the case actually occurred. On the other hand, if it occurred, it poses several grave problems. First, the practioner had not seen the patient previously, so no real patient/physician relationship had been established. Second, the physician chose to interpret the words of the patient to constitute a request for assisted euthanasia, which may or may not have been her intent. Third, the physician was morally obligated to discuss other clinical options, such as hospice, which assigns a high priority to the relief of pain and suffering. Fourth, other medications might have been used that avoided the suppression of respiration, while allowing the patient pain relief and rest. Fifth, a decision of such a devastatingly permanent nature is not one that should be taken without consultation. Given all these problems, the physician's actions could not have held up under the legal standard of basic common sense, and it is unlikely that if the physician had gone to court for this incident he would have been treated as lightly as Hans Florian or Bertram Harper.

Unfortunately there has been a cluster of cases involving nurses and mercy killing. Cases in California, Michigan, Texas, Florida, Maryland, Georgia, New York, and North Carolina have all made national headlines.[15] Most of these cases came to the attention of authorities as clusters of patient deaths and were detected in quality-assurance and risk-management studies. The impact upon the communities, the patient's families, and the nursing profession have been profound and negative. The intensity of the negative public reaction is perhaps a measure of how comfortable the average citizen is with the nurse as a patient advocate. When that trust is betrayed, there is a natural sense of outrage, as the "good nurse couldn't possibly act this way."

Mercy killing as an accepted practice is not something that can be entered into lightly, inasmuch as the act of putting someone to death—regardless of motive—involves the closure of all future options. It rules out any possibility of unanticipated discovery of wrong diagnosis, new treatments, spontaneous remission, or improvement as a result of continued treatment. There seems some right reasoning in the caution for prudence, "When in doubt - don't!"

ARGUMENTS FOR AND AGAINST EUTHANASIA

The arguments for the practice of euthanasia can be expressed in both utilitarian and duty-oriented terms. In the first case, it can be argued as a concern and compassion for those who are painfully and/or terminally ill. This view is strongly put forward by the noted ethicist and theologian Joseph Fletcher who feels that

> It is harder morally to justify letting someone die a slow and ugly death, dehumanized, than it is to justify helping him to escape from such misery. This is a case at least in any code of ethics which is humanististic or personalistic, i.e., in any code of ethics which has a value system that puts humanness and personal integrity above biological life and function.[16]

The duty-oriented arguments are centered on an extension of personal autonomy—the rights accorded us in western societies to live our life according to our own vision, unrestricted by the views of others. If we can live our lives according to a personal inner vision, then should this aspect of human dignity based on free choice also be extended to the termination of our lives? In Figure 8–4, the ethicist Arthur Dyck proposes a set of beliefs and propositions suitable as an ethic for euthanasia.[17]

For those who oppose active euthanasia on religious grounds, the basic concern seems to be the view that our lives are not ours but gifts from God. In this view, humans hold their lives as a trust. If this is true, then we are bound to hold not only the lives of others inviolate but also our own, since to take our life is to destroy what

An Ethic of Euthanasia

1. An individual's life belongs to that individual to dispose of entirely as he or she wishes;

2. The dignity that attaches to personhood by reason of the freedom to make choices demands also the freedom to take one's own life;

3. There is such a thing as life not worth living whether the cause be distress, illness, physical mental handicaps, or even sheer despair for whatever reason;

4. What is supreme in value is the human dignity that resides in the human's rational capacity to choose and control life and death.[17]

FIGURE 8-4

belongs to God. In Exodus 34:7 and Daniel 13:53, scriptures taken from the Old Testament, the doctrine of the sanctity of life principle is upheld, except in rare instances of self defense. Judeo-Christian precepts generally condemn active euthanasia in any form, but allow some forms of passive euthanasia. The difference is that of omission and commission: While the Judeo-Christian philosophy might tolerate the allowance of death, acts that *permit* death, it draws the line in regard to acts that *cause* death.

Nonreligious arguments against active euthanasia usually follow a slippery slope or wedge line of reasoning. In some ways the arguments recall the parable of the camel who pleaded with his owner to be allowed to put his nose into the tent to keep it warm against the cold desert night. Once the nose was allowed, other adjustments were requested, and the owner found himself sleeping with his camel. Is there something so persuasive about putting others to death that, if allowed, would become gross and commonplace? The Nazi "final solution," which brought about the death of millions of Jews, Gypsies, and other eastern Europeans, could be traced to compulsory euthanasia legislation that, at the time of its enactment, included only mental cases, monstrosities, and incurables that were a burden of the state. Using the Nazi experience as a guide, critics of active euthanasia do see some seductiveness to killing that humans do not seem able to handle. Perhaps Sigmund Freud was right as he wrote:[18]

> What no human soul desires there is no need to prohibit; it is automatically excluded. The very emphasis of the commandment "Thou shalt not kill" makes it certain that we spring from an endless ancestry of murderers, with whom the lust for killing was in the blood, as possibly it is to this day with ourselves.

The ethicist Joseph Fletcher feels that the use of the Nazi experience to show that a people can be taken down a primrose path, from a position of voluntary active euthanasia based on compassion and concern for human dignity to the grossness of the final solution, is too great a reach and is based on a false premise. He feels that what occurred in regard to the Nazi experience is not a slippery slope or wedge situation at all but rather an extension of the cruelty and lack of compassion built into the system at its very beginning. The Nazis did not go from mercy killing to the final solution, rather they started with merciless killing and proceeded from there. The Nazis did not fall into their practices on the basis of some fundamental seductiveness of killing. They began their practice through an acceptance of their bringing about the ends of the state through the involuntary control of its citizens.

Clearly, there is a wide chasm between the grossness of the actions of certain totalitarian states and the perceived need for voluntary euthanasia in the context of an American medical-moral-legal framework. The chasm is so wide that the use of the Nazi, Soviet, and Cambodian experiences is perhaps not suitable at all.

Yet, there is a need to look at the Netherlands experience to see if the lowering of the sanctity of life barriers leads to abuse. If euthanasia becomes too user friendly, are we setting the stage for abuser-friendly death? The Dutch government released a report indicating that, in a nation where 130,000 people die each year, there were annually about 5,000 to 10,000 cases of voluntary euthanasia. Some experts have extrapolated from the Dutch euthanasia experience that, if the same tolerance for the practice were adopted here, that might represent 75,000 to 150,000 voluntary euthanasia deaths per year. The report also estimated that in Holland there were probably another 1,000 unreported cases in which the physician brought about the deaths of patients without an explicit request from the patient to do so. The Dutch government reported that, in the decisions to terminate life without an explicit request, the physicians listed the following as important considerations, 31 percent, "low quality of life," 32 percent, "the family could not take it." In his book *Regulating Death: Euthanasia and the Case of the Netherlands,* Carlos Gomez writes:

> Throughout my study and analysis of the situation in the Netherlands, I have been plagued with the sense that something other than an argument for autonomy was at work. I have had the sense that some (physicians) felt that certain patients were better off dead, that it was a humane act to kill them.[19]

The question must be, "humane for whom?" Does our subjective view taken from a position of health, in regard to the quality of another's life, or how a family is suffering, justify the ending of a patient's life without his consent? Does the authority to kill an innocent individual provide the wedge that breaks down the barriers needed to protect the severely handicapped, unwanted newborns, the frail elderly, the "useless" members of our society? Once euthanasia is allowed and accepted, where is the rational ground upon which to stand and declare, "this far and no more!" Perhaps the rational ground called for by Carlos Gomez is clear and convincing evidence of the will of the individual patient, and where that is not provided or possible there can be no allowance for outside interference with life.

THE HOSPICE ALTERNATIVE

It is unlikely that the increased public acceptance of active euthanasia is based on any perceived need for an extension of personal autonomy to a "right to die." It is more likely that the genesis for the support is the fear of a lingering and painful death, surrounded by impersonal technicians, in a cold and unfamiliar environment.

If this is true then the resurgent **hospice movement** may make some arguments in regard to active euthanasia moot. The word hospice has been used since medieval times to indicate a place of rest for the weary traveler. In the modern usage of the term, the journey is different but the concept of rest and comfort are retained. The best-known hospice is St. Christopher's, in Great Britain, founded by Dr. Cicely Saunders in 1967. There are none of the usual trappings of a modern hospital. The rooms are cheerful, flowers are abundant, and the patients receive personalized care designed to virtually eliminate pain and suffering. Great effort is devoted to keeping the patient clean, caring for the skin, preventing bed sores, controlling nausea and vomiting, and treating neuropsychiatric symptoms. For the patient who is terminally ill, the balance between minimizing pain and suffering and the potential for hastening death is clearly struck in favor of relief of pain and suffering. Families are encouraged to stay all day and take their meals with the patients. Dying persons, when possible, are encouraged to take home visits whenever their stamina allows for them. The physicians and staff do not make rounds in white coats, ordering this and that, but rather there is a lot of touching, and hand-holding and listening. The emphasis is on honest communication with both the patients and their family. The dying patient is freed from as much pain as possible and encouraged to face the situation of death with dignity. For dying patients, the need for **palliative care** to relieve pain and suffering may rival the intensity of curative efforts found in the acute hospital setting.

Hospice programs are set up to provide palliative care, abatement of pain, and an environment that encourages dignity, but they do not cure or treat intensively. Pain suppression at this moment in medical practice is not absolute. There is no sure way to guarantee absolute freedom from pain or the side effects of modern medication. A final problem with the programs is their current lack of availability; there are many more patients who need the services than local facilities to support them. Since its inception, the hospice has ceased to be a place and has become a concept. Individual hospices now come in a variety of forms: community volunteer programs, home services, free-standing units, inhospital palliative care units, inhospital hospice teams, or combinations of each. In these cases, it is important for all health care providers to set a tone of caring and support. It is not the technology found in the hospital setting that dehumanizes, it is the human component or lack thereof. The basic philosophy of hospice is that dying is a natural part of life. The first two NHO standards are: "Appropriate therapy is the goal of hospice care," and "palliative care is the most appropriate care when cure is no longer possible."[20]

The hospice concept has been very effective in dealing with the terminally ill. These are specialized units designed to reduce suffering and provide humane care for the dying. The hospice movement, while developed in England, has blossomed in the United States—largely through the encouragement of Dr. Elisabeth Kübler-Ross.

SUMMARY

In the United States, the practice of passive euthanasia for the terminally ill and in limited cases for those who persist in a chronic vegetative state has generally been accepted by the courts and health care practitioners. Under special circumstances, health care providers have found it ethically permissible to omit further life-extending technology and to allow patients to die. Given that the end results appear to be the same for passive and active euthanasia, many advocates of euthanasia have petitioned for the broadening of the practice to include the more active forms wherein health care practitioners could assist in hastening the dying process. Active euthanasia, which includes mercy killing, is currently forbidden under law and by all professional codes of health care ethics in the United States.

The practice of active euthanasia has been tolerated in the Netherlands for over a decade but it has only recently been legalized. Although it is illegal in the United States, polls indicate a shift of public opinion to favor the practice of active euthanasia. The highly publicized Quinlan, Cruzan, and Bouvia cases coupled with the activities of such groups as the Hemlock Society have brought the issue to a level of public awareness that makes its legalization a distinct possibility in the next decade. The major concerns of those favoring the adoption of active euthanasia appear to be the fear of a painful lingering death as well as the desire to further the principle of personal autonomy to include a right to die.

It is clear that modern health care delivery as it addresses the end of life is a frightening consideration for many Americans. The thought of cold sterile rooms, filled with cold professionals, invasive tubes and instruments, lingering unconsciousness, and great financial burden all seem part of this new way of dying. Our health care policies often make the elderly spend down to poverty in order to access the care they need, in the end leaving a surviving spouse destitute. If these are the factors that have lead to the great interest in euthanasia, then would it be as appealing if the dying process were less cold and terrible? The answer may lie in reforming a broken system rather than ushering in the obiatrist.

The increased availability of hospice centers may offer some relief for terminally ill patients who fear a painful lingering death, isolated from loved ones, and surrounded by cold technology and technocrats. These centers specialize in palliative care where patients are allowed to come to grips with their mortality, and to prepare themselves for death.

Those who oppose the acceptance of active euthanasia within health care do so generally using two lines of reasoning. First, there are those who oppose active euthanasia on the basis of the principle of sanctity of life. All life in this sense has infinite value, and therefore any portion of life also has infinite value, whether that be 10 minutes or 10 years. Others base their opposition on the feeling that allowing assisted euthanasia for the terminally ill might be the start of a slippery slope or a beginning wedge philosophy that, once begun, could lead to extermination of the elderly or the malformed.

The argument that allowing one kind of justifiable action could conceivably increase the tendency to allow another kind of unjustified action seems somewhat spurious, unless there is a natural tendency toward the second type of action. If adopted, the slippery slope argument could easily be used to avoid any new thinking and defend the status quo in all areas of our lives.

Whatever the convictions of health care providers, they should follow the current arguments in regard to euthanasia closely. Currently, in all jurisdictions within the United States, active euthanasia is illegal and considered homicide. In the near future this might change, at which time our current codes of ethics will need to be rethought and modified if assisted death becomes legal, as in the Netherlands.

CLARIFICATION EXERCISES

A. In Shakespeare's *Julius Caesar,* Brutus asks his friend Volumnius to assist him in death, after he has suffered defeat in battle.

> Thou seest the world, Volumnius, how it goes;
> Our enemies have beat us to the pit:
> It is more worthy to leap in ourselves,
> Than tarry till they push us, Good Volumnius,
> Thou know'st that we two went to school together;
> Even for that our love of old, I prithee,
> Hold thou my sword-hilts whilst I run on it.
>
> Volumnius replies, "That's not an office for a friend,
> My Lord.

One reason often given not to continue further down the path of active euthanasia and to adopt it as a practice by health care workers is similar to that offered by Volumnius. "Putting individuals to death is not an office of a health care provider." In her article, "Where Do You Stand on Euthanasia?" Amy Haddad [21] argues that active euthanasia would harm the nursing profession, as patients currently see nurses as nurturing, compassionate patient advocates. Would their participation in death inducement place their role as nurses at risk?

B. In 1921, George Minot, at the age of 36, was found to have diabetes. Following the current medical practice of his time he attempted to control his disease by diet; however it was obvious that he was fighting a losing battle. In 1923, insulin became available, reversed his disease, and saved his life. Minot went on with his research, and in 1927, reported that the ingestion of large amounts of liver could bring about regeneration of red cells in the bone marrow. This became the first effective treatment for pernicious anemia and won for Minot the 1934 Nobel prize.

This anecdote is often used by those who oppose both active and passive euthanasia on the basis "Suppose a cure is found?" Respond to the argument of the miraculous cure.

C. The David Letterman show has used the Kevorkian suicide machine ("the thanatron") as a source of at least two of its "Top Ten" comedy lists. One listed the following among Top Ten promotional slogans for the device.

> "Claus von Bulow says 'I liked it so much I bought the company!'"
> "While I'm killing myself, I'm also cleaning my oven!"
> "Isn't it about time you took an honest look at your miserable, stinking life?"

The final quote points to a real problem with lowering the barriers to active euthanasia. How do we screen for those patients who do not particularly wish to die but are only depressed at the moment? Most terminally ill or frail elderly have periods of severe depression in which they might request active euthanasia one day and regret it the next. Popular publications such as *Final Exit*"[22] are little more than "how to" books and deal with emotions such as depression in a very light manner. One could imagine a person suffering from depression using the book as a suicide manual. Assuming that we have decided to allow active euthanasia, what rules would you put into place to protect against its improper usage? Create five such rules:

D. Current diagnostics allow mothers to find out a great deal of information in regard to the unborn. In cases where the tests show severe genetic problems, often the woman is counseled regarding abortion. Is this a form of euthanasia?

E. Due to our general acceptance of the rule of law in our society, we might hear the argument that we should not practice euthanasia because it is an illegal act. Is this an ethical argument? Defend your answer.

F. It is clear that having individuals report to a van hidden in a county park (as did Kevorkian) in order to be assisted in dying is untenable. However, equally untenable is the treatment of Hans Florian and Bertram Harper, who faced trial for assisting loved ones in death. Kevorkian has suggested setting up "Obitoriums" for suicide seekers, with trained specialists to perform the services. What safeguards would you want put into place to protect the system from becoming a method by which society gets rid of the weak and undesirable? List four. (For example, "No one can be sent to Obiatry without the recommendation of two doctors, one of whom may not be previously involved in your care.)

G. Grandpa's Grandpa (GG for short) was to die tomorrow, but three members of the family couldn't get away for the funeral, so the time was postponed again, giving him his sixth new lease on life. GG died once, but at the time he was in the large tertiary hospital having surgery, so when his heart stopped they hooked him to an artificial heart and restored his life. That was more than fifty years ago, and the doctors and nurses involved are gone now.

Actually, considering his 125 years, GG is in good shape, and with social security, Medicare, and such he is no burden. He only weighs 90 pounds, so it doesn't cost much to feed him; and in that he sits very still, his clothes last a long time, although as time passes they do go out of style.

When I was born, the family decided not to replace his battery and, therefore, have a June funeral. I understand that the decision didn't come easy, and took most of the afternoon. Much of the opposition to letting GG die arose from the fact that he was in really good shape for a man his age. His heart was good; only his mind had run down. By a slim majority, GG was doomed, but then he was resurrected because someone noted that the decision could not be made without a quorum present.

GG's funeral did not come up again for years—not so much because his health got better, but because he was beginning to have fewer relatives. Perhaps the decision to allow him to die was postponed because the small amount of money he had invested had grown to a tidy sum, and the closest relative was a no-good nephew who didn't deserve the money, or so mom and dad said. The vote was to keep GG with us, and farsighted it was, as the no-good nephew died the next year. With the no-good gone, there seemed little reason to prolong the old gentleman's life, so a special family meeting was called. GG had become a little more forgetful and had at times skipped meals. Before the matter was decided, two of the junior members, who were pre-med students, said that they thought GG should be preserved as a geriatric model. The logic of their argument won the day and GG was allowed to live.

Later that week, GG broke his leg and was sent to a hospital, where the doctors and nurses began to debate the issue. Merely removing the stimulus to the heart could not be considered murder, they argued, as the heart God gave him was still in there. If they removed the stimulus and the heart stopped, it became God's will.

A meeting of the clan was called, as it was felt that only the family could make such a decision. This fifth make-or-break decision was complicated by the fact that a new device had just been invented and, if installed, would prolong GG's life indefinitely, possibly for hundreds of years. This new twist to the GG problem completely destroyed the decision-making system. No decision was made, as three family members said that they couldn't make it to a funeral, although we all knew they really could.[22]

In all ethical cases it is useful to attempt to ascertain the effects of motivation on decision making. Examine the rather fanciful case of GG and answer the following questions.

1. Who were the main parties with interests in the outcome for GG?

2. What might be the options selected as a final solution? List three.

3. What might be the motivations of the following individuals, given each of your three options?
   GG
   Family
   Health Care Providers

H. Write five value statements that fit your beliefs about active euthanasia as a medical practice.

REFERENCES AND SUGGESTED READING

1. Jack Kevorkian, *Prescription: Medicide* (Buffalo: Prometheus Books, 1991), 231.
2. Jack Kevorkian, *Prescription: Medicide*.
3. Jack Kevorkian, *Prescription: Medicide*, p. 228.

4. Ronald Munson, *Intervention and Reflection: Basic Issues in Medical Ethics* (Belmont, CA: Wadsworth Publishing Co., 1983), 142.

5. Bob Richards, Palos Verdes Estates, CA, Poem dedicated to the staff of Harbor General Hospital, Torrence CA.

6. Tom Beauchamp, "What Is Suicide? in *Ethical Issues in Death and Dying,* eds. T. Beauchamp and P. Seymour (Englewood Cliffs, NJ: Prentice Hall, 1978), 97–102.

7. Jack Kevorkian, *Medicide,* p. 196.

8. Arthur Caplan, "Disabled Women Are Victimized by Kevorkian" *Detroit Free Press,* 9 June, 1992, p. 2C.

9. *Notre Dame Lawyer* 48 (1973):1202–1260.

10. Marcia Angell, "Euthanasia," *The New England Journal of Medicine* 319, no. 20 (November 17, 1988): 1348–1350.

11. Andrew Greeley, "Live and Let Die: Changing Attitudes," *The Christian Century* (4 December, 1991): 1124–1125.

12. James Rachels, *The End of Life* (Oxford: Oxford University Press, 1986).

13. Betty DeRamus, "Without a Clear Law, We Can't Point Fingers at Assisted Suicide," *The Detroit News* (Sunday, October 1991).

14. Name Withheld, "It's Over, Debbie" *Journal of the American Medical Association* 259(2) (1988): 272.

15. Beatrice Yorker, "Nurses Accused of Murder," *American Journal of Nursing* (October 1988): 1327–1332.

16. Joseph Fletcher, "The Right to Live and the Right to Die," *The Humanist* 34 (4) (1974).

17. Arthur Dyck, "An Alternative to the Ethic of Euthanasia," in *To Live and Die, When, Why and How,* R. Williams, ed. (New York: Springer-Verlag, 1974).

18. Sigmund Freud, "Thoughts for the Times on War and Death, 1915," in *Collected Papers,* Vol. IV (London: Hogarth Press, 1925).

19. Carlos Gomez, *Regulating Death: Euthanasia and the Case of the Netherlands* (New York: The Free Press, 1991).

20. National Hospice Organization, Standards and Accreditation Committee, *Standards of a Hospice Program* (Mclean, VA, 1979).

21. Amy Haddad, "Where Do You Stand On Euthanasia" *RN* (April 1991): 43.

22. Derek Humphry, *Final Exit* (Eugene, OR: The Hemlock Society, 1991).

23. Robert Francoeur, *Biomedical Ethics* (New York: Wiley Medical Publications, 1983).

CHAPTER 9

Abortion

Instructional Goal

The general goal of this chapter is to outline the nature of the conflict between the pro-life (anti-abortion) position and the pro-choice position (not necessarily pro-abortion, but against legislation outlawing abortion).

Instructional Objectives

At the end of this chapter the reader should understand and be able to:

1. Outline the distinction between *"human"* and *"person,"* and the dispute regarding personhood criteria.
2. Describe the distinction between the quality of life and life itself.
3. List the basic facts of fetal development.
4. Describe the sociology of the abortion issue.
5. Outline the religious arguments against abortion.
6. Argue the issue of rights from a utilitarian understanding.
7. List the difficulties with arguments based on self-defense.
8. List the elements of the doctrine of double-effect and state when it is used.
9. Outline the significance of Thomson's analogies.
10. List the Freedom of Religion arguments.
11. Explain the pro-choice position from a "life plan" point of view.
12. State how the power of sexuality is involved in the abortion issue.
13. State how an environmental perspective might affect your understanding of the abortion issue.
14. Explain how issues of civil disobedience are involved in the politics of abortion.
15. Explain the different types of abortion.

Glossary

Conceptus (single-celled zygote): The union of a spermatozoon and an ovum, which occurs at conception.

Double Effect: When an action has more than one consequence.

Embryo: Between two and three weeks into pregnancy and until the eighth week the identification of the zygote as implanted into the uterine wall.

Fetus: The term used from the time when brain waves can be monitored (beginning in the eighth week) until birth at nine months.

Necessary Condition: A circumstance that must be present for something to occur.

Norplant: "The underarm pill," a long-lasting implant for women that prevents pregnancy for five years.

Ovum: The female germ cell.

Person: A living entity with moral standing, possibly a right to life (not necessarily equivalent to "human").

Quickening: The point at which the mother feels the fetus move.

RU 486: "The abortion pill," which causes a woman to spontaneously abort.

Speciesism: Discrimination based solely on one's membership in a species.

Spermatozoon: The male germ cell.

Sufficient Condition: A circumstance that will bring about the occurrence of something else.

Viability: The stage at which the fetus can live independent of the mother's body.

Zygote (multi-celled zygote): Comes into being in first 24 hours with the splitting of the conceptus and continues until the zygote becomes implanted into the uterine wall.

THE ABORTION ISSUE

What is an abortion? There are two common techniques that are referred to as abortions. One is **uterine** or **vacuum aspiration,** in which the cervix is widened by instruments, a tube is inserted into the uterus, and its contents are suctioned out. The other method is called **dilation and curettage.** The method is the same except that, instead of using suction, the contents of the uterus are scraped out with the use of a surgical instrument. Late abortions, which are less common, are brought about through the use of a saline injection, which induces a miscarriage. Although rarely used, cesarean sections are also sometimes used to abort a fetus.

The abortion issue is a highly contested one, and it is likely to become even more explosive. *Roe v. Wade,* the Supreme Court case that legalized abortion in the United States, has been under attack for years. The law still stands, in spite of the fears of those who thought the Reagan and Bush appointees to the Supreme Court would overturn it, but abortion laws have been passed across the country, and civil disobedience, harassment, and vandalism are increasingly prevalent as more traditional methods of changing laws and minds have been exhausted. It is into this highly emotional arena that we now enter.

The Legal Issues

The *Roe v. Wade* Supreme Court decision of 1973 was based essentially on a right to privacy, but it restricted the right by splitting pregnancies into three "trimesters," with personal liberty restricted as the pregnancy enters the third trimester.

The first trimester is a period of personal liberty. The woman is free to abort the fetus at her own discretion.

In the second trimester of pregnancy the state may restrict the abortion procedure in ways reasonably related to maternal health.

During the third trimester, the state may regulate or even prohibit abortion, except in cases where the life or health of the mother is in danger.

The reasoning behind the Roe decision was based on a right to privacy. Critics of *Roe* argue that there is no basis for a right to privacy in the Constitution. Who is right? One's position on the right to privacy is related to one's theory of constitutional interpretation. There are many schools of legal interpretation, but two of the most influential are "original intent" and what we will call the "progressivist" interpretation. Followers of original intent argue that the U.S. Constitution is to be interpreted according to what likely was the intent of the authors of the Constitution. The Constitution is seen as a monumental document to a short-lived rule of reason in 1776. Progressivists, on the other hand, argue that the tenth Amendment to the Constitution, which says that the enumeration of certain rights does not exclude the existence of others, is conclusive. The progressivist sees the Constitution as a living document linked to the increasing understanding of the concept of freedom.

Some argue that we are wrong to look to the Supreme Court to resolve the issue. After all, couldn't we resolve this state by state? Or couldn't Congress just pass a law one way or another? Presidents Reagan and Bush used the power of the presidency to further the pro-life agenda, and Clinton, in turn, is in favor of switching the laws back to the pro-choice side. In 1994 this means that the pro-choice side wins; in 1996 or 2001, who knows? The problem with executive orders, however, is that they can be overturned by executive order. Congress may be the place to make the decision because it is most closely in touch with the will of the people, and because its decisions tend to be long-lived. All in all, there does not seem to be any appropriate arena for deciding how the law should read. The fact that the two sides cannot seem to get a secure and long-term grip on legislation may indicate that we should go back to the philosophical drawing board—which may be a good thing anyway.

It is important to realize that even if the legal issue were resolved, the question of whether abortion is a *moral* issue would remain. If any side is to "win," it should be by force of the better moral argument, not because of what someone might have meant over 200 years ago or because the votes have moved left or right this week.

The Moral Issues

The abortion issue involves many of the same concepts that underlie the issues of euthanasia and impaired infants. In each of these issues, there are disputes concerning personhood, sanctity of life, quality of life, autonomy, and mercy—as well as larger concepts such as freedom and social stability. The health care professional is often placed in situations that involve adjudicating among these concepts, and more often is placed in situations in which others make decisions using these concepts. The fact that others make these decisions does not mean the health care professional can ignore them, for he or she is often put in the position of carrying out the decisions. So even if one has no role in the decision-making process, one may need to come to terms with actions that may be morally controversial and emotionally heartrending.

The Two Positions

The pro-life position: Anti-abortion, believes abortion is murder and should be stopped.

The pro-choice position: Believes that the decision to abort is one of personal liberty and thus should be legal.

There are two possible subpositions:

1. One may believe that abortion is wrong but, for whatever reason, is something that should be up to every individual to decide. The issue becomes an individual or "personal" decision.
2. One may believe there is nothing wrong with abortion or that, while abortion is wrong, it can be outweighed by other considerations.

The Sanctity of Life Argument

The first argument we will discuss is that against abortion based on the sanctity of life. The argument states that since the fetus is alive it is sacred and must therefore not be killed. This argument is not persuasive as it stands, for we kill many entities that are alive; indeed we must, for nutrition requires that we at least eat plants, and plants are surely alive. The argument is then usually revised so that it begins with the claim that all human life is sacred. It is sometimes presented by referring to the human genetic code. The argument claims that since the full genetic code of a human being is present at conception, then a human life begins at that point as well; thus, abortion should not be permitted.

The Genetic Code Argument

Some argue that having a genetic code of a human being is not sufficient to establish humanity. It is argued that, just as an acorn is not an oak, nor a three-year-old a man, neither is a fetus a human being. This dispute raises the question: Does the potential for becoming human give an entity the same rights as a human being?

After all, one must first be a fetus to be a human. On the other hand, we often distinguish the rights of people based on age. A twelve-year-old does not have the right to drive although she certainly has the potential to do so when she is older. Nor do minors have the right to drink, smoke cigarettes, or see X-rated movies. The question is whether the right to life is such a right. Does the right to life come into existence with conception?

There is another problem with the genetic code argument. Down syndrome babies do not have the same genetic structure as normal human beings; in fact, it is the cause of their condition. Does this mean they do not have a right to life? The same argument would apply to extraterrestrials if we should happen to encounter any. They would surely not be human; does that mean they would not have a right to life? The antiabortionist could respond, however, that a human genetic code is a sufficient but not a necessary condition of beings with a right to life. Thus, other entities may have a right to life, but it is argued that an entity with a human genetic code definitely has such a right.

The Facts of Fetal Development

The next set of issues requires some discussion of the facts of fetal development. The union of the sperm and egg gives us what is called a **conceptus.** As we have pointed out, there is already a full genetic code such that the sex, hair color, skin color, and various other attributes are already determined. We encounter a problem when we consider the stage of development, the **zygote,** which comes into being in the first 24 hours. The problem is this: It is still not determined whether there is a single human, twins, triplets, or whatever. How can we say there is a human if we don't know how many there are? One might respond by saying that, however many there are, whatever is there is a human. So if there are two, there are two humans. But this is not quite good enough, for the zygote sometimes splits and then reunites. Are we to say that what is one human becomes two and then one again?

Two to three weeks into the pregnancy the zygote settles into the uterine wall and the possible twins problem is resolved. At this stage, the entity is called an **embryo.** No special problems arise at this stage for the abortion argument, but some pro-choice theorists point out that we still do not have anything that looks remotely human. The embryo looks like it has a tail and gills. Nor do the rudimentary eyes, ears, kidneys, or liver work yet. Pro-life theorists counter that we should not base our moral judgments upon looks, and they point to the history of racism as a case where basing moral worth on appearance has had horrendous consequences.

At eight weeks we call the entity a **fetus,** which it will remain until birth. We will also use this term for the entity from conception to birth unless the argument requires a more specific term. In the third month the fetus starts to move, and by the fourth month the mother can feel the movement. The point at which the mother can sense the fetus moving is called **quickening.** It was once believed that the fetus gained a soul at this stage, but since it does not really coincide with any major medical changes most tend to disregard quickening as important to the abortion issue. By the fifth month, the fetus can feel pain and is therefore due the same consideration we would give to other creatures that can feel pain. In the sixth month, the fetus becomes viable, and by the seventh the fetus has neurons that are developed enough for a minimal consciousness.

Birth generally occurs after nine months, but the baby is still completely dependent on the mother, or at least some mother. Anti-abortion theorists argue that there is no real medical change, so those who would grant only the newborn a right to life are left to come up with an argument that would justify a right to life for a newborn but not a fetus five minutes before birth. Since the changes are so gradual throughout the development of the fetus, it is difficult to point to a stage that clearly separates a human from a pre-human.

Killing and Self-Defense

Up to this point we have assumed that killing is always wrong. But it is not true that all killing of human beings is impermissible, for there is a widely accepted exception: self-defense. If someone is about to kill you, and the only way to save yourself is to kill the other person first, then killing is permissible, at least for most people. Some believe that this means we should allow abortions when the mother's life is in danger. Others point out that killing in self-defense is only permissible when your attacker is intentionally trying to kill you. You may not, for example, kill an innocent person who threatens your life by accident. One cannot shove an innocent person in front of a speeding car in order to save oneself.

The problem with the moral assessment of such actions arises from what we may call the "multiple character" of most actions. When I turn on a light, I am not only providing illumination to a room; I may also be signaling an accomplice, testing the electricity, or any number of things. One attempt to come to terms with such complex actions—actions that have more than one meaning and/or consequence—focuses on the "multiple" character of human action. The doctrine of double effect comes to us from the philosopher, St. Thomas Aquinas. The doctrine asks us to distinguish the intended effect of an action from other, unintended effects. This doctrine has been used to justify the death of fetuses under certain circumstances that threaten the life of the mother. Ovarian cancer sometimes must be treated with a full hysterectomy, and such an operation results in the death of the fetus. Note that the intention here is to save the mother, not to kill the fetus. Note also that it would be impermissible, according to this doctrine, to perform an abortion to save a mother from death if the procedure involved the direct killing of the fetus. It is only permissible if the death of the fetus is an indirect cause of the death of the fetus.

"Human" or "Person"?

Mary Anne Warren has argued for a distinction between "human" and "person."[1] While one is human by virtue of one's genetic code, a **person** is a member of the moral community. One becomes a member of the moral community by having certain characteristics recognized by the community as grounded in moral status and, in particular, rights. There are various characteristics that might qualify one for personhood. The following list of traits central to personhood are worth consideration:

1. Consciousness of objects and events
2. The ability to feel pain
3. Reasoning
4. Self-motivated activity
5. The capacity to communicate
6. A concept of the self [2]

While one may differ about one or more members of this list, it does seem to capture most people's understanding of personhood. If an entity were not conscious (permanently; it is not permissible to kill people when they are asleep), it would be difficult to summon any objection to injuring such an entity.

The same goes for the ability to feel pain. However, the other characteristics are more controversial. What sort of reasoning do we have in mind? A dog who chooses one direction over another at a fork in the road is using some sort of reasoning. Do we wish to include dogs as persons? Some animal rights theorists make the odd but possibly valid argument that some adult mammals have rights while human fetuses do not. Notice also that injured humans who can no longer reason are not persons under this criterion either. The important point is that it is difficult to pose criteria that include fetuses but not animals, that exclude animals and permanently comatose humans without also excluding fetuses.

What about self-motivated activity? It is difficult to imagine any being having moral standing that did not direct its own actions or at least have the motivation to do so. On the other hand, one might argue that, as long as it feels pain, then it should not feel pain needlessly if it is innocent.

The requirement that an entity be able to communicate is a rather stringent one. Newborns cannot really communicate, so if this were a necessary condition of personhood, even infanticide would be permissible. Some philosophers, such as Michael Tooley[3] have taken the position that infanticide is permissible because newborns have no concept of self. Tooley is thinking primarily of defective newborns; nevertheless, it is clear that the last two criteria are problematic.

One might object to the practice of listing characteristics of personhood altogether. After all, the idea of restricting moral standing to only those humans with certain characteristics has led in the past to racism, sexism, and religious intolerance. But one might also argue that historically the problem has been that race, sex, and religious affiliation have not matched up with any rational division of entities. The problem, then, is not having criteria but having bad criteria. Note that adult humans of any race, sex, or religious affiliation do meet the above criteria. Furthermore, unless we are to be **speciesist** and arbitrarily assign moral standing to humans, we must come up with criteria for personhood. One can imagine, after all, that we will someday encounter aliens that are clearly not possessed of a human genetic code and upon whom we may wish to confer personhood.

Warren does not argue that personhood requires all of the above characteristics. The first three or four would probably be sufficient. What we should note is the fact that a conceptus meets none of the criteria. The earliest possible point that a fetus could feel pain would be at eight weeks, when brain activity becomes detectable, since feeling pain involves brain activity. This does not mean that an eight-week-old fetus can feel pain; eight weeks is the earliest date at which pain would be possible. The other characteristics generally do not manifest themselves until after birth.

The Viability Argument

Another criterion for personhood not mentioned by Warren, **viability,** focuses on the characteristic of biological independence. Some argue that a fetus has standing only when it becomes viable outside the mother. The idea is that personhood requires some sort of independence from other people, particularly the mother. Since the fetus has standing only as a dependent on the mother, it follows that the mother has the last word on whether it comes to viability. Once viability is achieved, however, the mother no longer has exclusive say over the fetus; indeed, the state might have a compelling interest in seeing to it that viable fetuses come to term. The reasoning is that once a fetus is viable it is no longer completely dependent on a particular mother, and therefore if others wish to take the burden from the original mother they should be allowed to do so. Given the numbers of people having difficulty adopting children, such an argument is not without merit. If another person wishes to take care of and raise a baby instead of its being aborted, it is hard to imagine anyone objecting.

The objection to using viability as a criterion for personhood is that it varies over time and place. What this means is that, as medical technology develops, what counts as a person will change. More troubling, still, is the fact that a fetus that would be a person in a major hospital in the United States but not in a developing country without sophisticated medical facilities. One wonders why the idea of a variable concept of personhood is so problematic. After all, personhood is not a natural property that one can discern like sodium in salt. It is a moral property, which means it is a matter of human decision whether or not to grant it to an entity. Furthermore, what is wrong with viability varying from place to place? People die all the time all over the world because of a lack of medical facilities. In fact, there is a certain sense to this sort of variability. In some places where infant mortality is high, personhood decisions are often postponed to up to three years of age, at which point the baby is given a name. Such a practice makes sense in the light of the emotional weight given to the loss of a child who is regarded as a person.

There are some philosophers who believe that there is more to the abortion question than the issue of personhood. Judith Thomson has argued that, even if we were to grant personhood to the fetus (which she is not willing to do), abortions may still be permissible.[4] Thomson uses the method of analogical thought experiments. She builds a scenario that leads us to the conclusion she wants. Then she shows us how our view on the abortion issue should follow the same reasoning. The method of analogy is very powerful, for it requires only our assent to consistency.

You will find these arguments outrageous as well as enlightening. The following arguments are worthwhile, if only as logic exercises, even if they fail to convince.

The Violinist Analogy. Thomson asks us to imagine a famous violinist whose kidneys are failing (Figure 9–1). The Society of Music Lovers, we are also asked to imagine, decides to kidnap you in the middle of the night and hook you up to the violinist for nine months or so until a kidney donor can be found. Thomson asks us whether we would feel obligated to remain hooked to the violinist for nine months or whether we would consider it morally permissible to unhook ourselves from the violinist. She anticipates that our answer will be that it is permissible to unhook ourselves because of our rights over our own bodies. The application to the abortion issue is clear. If it is morally permissible to unhook ourselves from the violinist, then, by the same reasoning, it must also be permissible to have an abortion, and this is true even if we regard the fetus as a person.

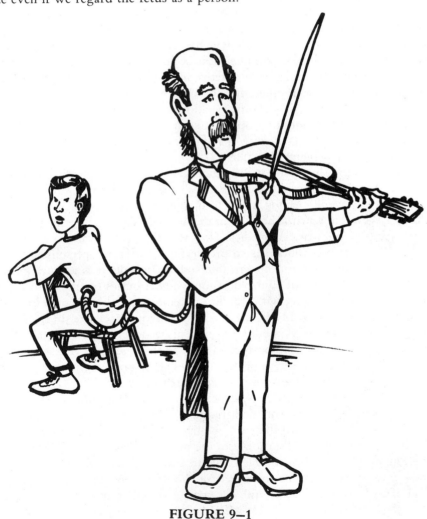

FIGURE 9–1

One might argue that there is a disanalogy involved, for pregnancy is not like a kidnapping. Rather, it is voluntary. Fair enough. However, what about the case of rape? Rape is, by definition, involuntary, yet many regard abortion in rape cases to be just as wrong as in voluntary pregnancies, since it is not the baby's fault it was brought about involuntarily. Such people must, therefore, agree to staying hooked to the violinist for nine months. Some are willing to "bite this bullet," but many others will find themselves in a contradictory position. Notice, though, that if we are not willing to bite the bullet we are then obligated to agree that there is at least one case when personhood may be overridden for other reasons. This is crucial, since it provides a wedge for the pro-choice person to slip an exception into the otherwise impregnable right to life of innocent persons. Once we accept this exception, so the reasoning goes, we will also be forced to accept others.

The Rapidly Growing Child Analogy. This analogy attempts to call attention to the case of abortion when the mother's life is in danger. Imagine yourself in a house with a rapidly growing child. In fact, the child is growing so rapidly that you find your exits blocked by the baby and on the verge of suffocation (Figure 9–2). The only way for you to survive is for you to kill the baby. Again, Thomson believes we will agree that killing an innocent is permissible in this case. Hence, we have another exception to the right to life of innocent persons. This case, like the one we have just

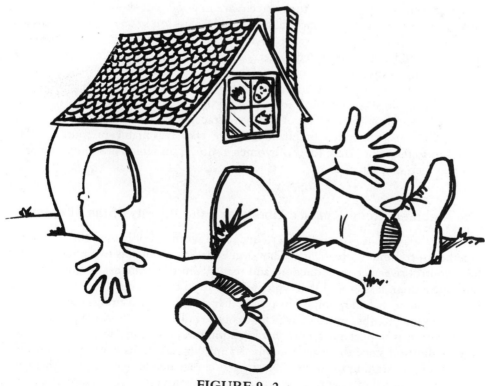

FIGURE 9–2

considered, has problems. Is it true that it is acceptable to kill innocent people in order to save ourselves? Consider another case. You find yourself caught in a flooding tunnel and the only exit is blocked by a fat man who is lodged in the exit. The water will eventually force him out, but you will have drowned by that time. Would you be within your rights if you used dynamite to dislodge and therefore kill the fat man? Many, if not most, would say that doing so is not permissible. The argument would be that it is only right to kill in self-defense, when the other person is intentionally trying to kill you. But this does not work either, for most would regard it as permissible to kill a deranged man in self-defense even though the person is not responsible for his insanity. The only thing clear here is that self-defense cases are far from morally unambiguous. What is interesting, in spite of the ambiguity of the reasoning behind self-defense, is that the vast majority of people regard saving the life of the mother a clear case of permissible abortion. There is a vocal minority, however, who would make distinctions between cases of danger to the mother's life, namely those enamored with the doctrine of double effect that we discussed earlier.

The Carpet-Seed Children Analogy. The final analogy we will borrow from Thomson is meant to call attention to the case of failed contraception. Imagine that, instead of the reproductive process being as we understand it, children are the result of airborne seeds that germinate in carpeting. We can imagine that people will be rather concerned to make sure their screens are in good working order. But we can also imagine that, in spite of such diligence, holes develop in one of our screens and some seeds germinate in our carpet. Are we obligated to bring these children to term, or would we be permitted to get the vacuum cleaner from the closet (Figure 9–3)? Thomson thinks that vacuuming should be permitted. The analogy, as we have indicated, is with faulty contraception.

If one is inclined to agree to vacuuming up the carpet-seed children, one should also agree to abortion in the case of faulty contraception. The idea is that we are not responsible for unintended pregnancies if we take reasonable precautions. This brings us to the rather large topic of women's choice, on which pro-choice theorists rest so much of their case.

The Argument from Women's Liberty and the Priority of the Lifeplan

For many women, it is unthinkable to imagine a woman not having the decision of whether to continue a pregnancy. They argue that if a woman is to be free she must have control over her reproduction, and that, given the immense responsibility of raising children, it is crucial that women be allowed to determine when it happens. Others counter that adoption is always another option, which brings the obligation down to nine months, much of which does not really interfere with a person's life. (However, it is important to note that adoption does not really work as an alternative to abortion since there are roughly 1.5 million abortions every year but only 50,000 couples waiting to adopt.) But the pro-choice person will respond that even this asks too much of a woman. If a woman is to compete in the marketplace with men, she cannot have pregnancy interrupting her career. To regard a woman's

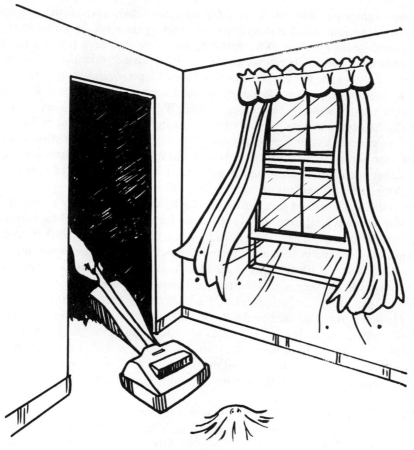

FIGURE 9–3

career—or more generally her lifeplan—as having so little importance that it must be set aside by the contingency of unwanted pregnancy is to regard women as less important than men. This is true whether the woman works at home or in the marketplace. What is crucial is that a woman have control over her lifeplan in the way a man has control. If your plan is to raise two children, then to impose a third is to violate the woman's right to choose the course of her life. This is what leads many women to say that if men became pregnant there would be no abortion controversy.

At this point, pro-life people argue that women can "just say no." Women do not have to engage in sex. In fact, it is argued that the root of the abortion problem is precisely the modern attitude toward sex. Notice that we are now in another area of intense and deep disagreement. What we find at this level of argument are differing ideas concerning sexuality, ideas that ultimately come down to one's religious or most deeply held moral beliefs. We will discuss this broad topic later in the chapter, for now we must point out that even married women want the choice as to the time of pregnancy. Are we to ask married women to refrain from sex? Isn't that asking rather too much?

Some might argue that we are making altogether too much of the possibility of failed contraception, and that if women were merely responsible with contraception there would be no problem. The problem with this argument is that even the pill sometimes fails, and further, many women either cannot take the pill at all or are advised not to take the pill longer than five years. Contraception other than the pill is rather less effective, and unwanted pregnancies are bound to happen. We must also remember what it is we are asking of people. We are asking that they act perfectly rationally in situations that we all know to bring out a great deal of irrationality. This is, of course, less of a problem the older we get, but the abortion issue is not one just for adults; it is one that is most tragic for minors. According to the Alan Guttmacher Institute, more than 25 percent of abortions are performed on teenagers. More than 60 percent are under 25.

It is in this light that we must understand why there are so many abortions. Take, for example, the typical first sexual experience for many children. Much of the time, intercourse is not on the evening's agenda, but as the night progresses things get too hot and heavy for many teenagers to resist. Since intercourse was not planned it is also unlikely that the teens thought ahead to bring contraceptives. Again, we must notice what we are asking of children: to behave with complete rationality in an unfamiliar situation in which their bodies' hormones are working against rationality. Now it is true that this problem can be somewhat overcome if we supply all teenagers with contraceptives, as well as sex education before they reach the age of sexuality. But many, if not most, abortion opponents would reject such practices as encouraging promiscuity. It is argued that, without the fear of pregnancy, teens will likely indulge in sex more often—with the added consequence of possibly contracting AIDS.

The phenomenon of AIDS is instructive, for it shows how powerful the urge to have sex really is. In spite of the threat of death, teens and even adults continue to have unprotected sex and sex with multiple partners. What this shows is that the threat of pregnancy is unlikely to act as an effective deterrent to sex, given that most people regard the threat of death as worse than pregnancy, and even the threat of death fails to deter. Some argue that people really have not come to terms with the reality that they are in mortal danger when they engage in unprotected sex, whereas they are very clear about the danger of pregnancy. One could respond by noting that the number of unwanted pregnancies shows that if we are in denial concerning the threat of AIDS, we are also in denial concerning pregnancy. In any case, we should not rely on the fear of pregnancy to play much of a role in preventing promiscuity.

We should also respond to the idea that "if you play, you pay." The idea here is that if you consent to sex and get pregnant, it is only just. This sort of vindictiveness has no place in moral philosophy, and it certainly makes no sense from the social point of view. Should we regard children as punishment? Some argue that the task of raising a child is too difficult and demanding to turn it over to someone who is regarded as irresponsible in the first place. No one believes that "babies should have babies"; the question is how to prevent it. Given the well-known cycle of poverty of underage, single mothers, the overriding social problem according to pro-choice theorists is teenage pregnancy, not abortion. The crucial question concerns our overall quality of life rather than biological existence. It is pointed out, for example, that 62 percent of the families of the women who have abortions have incomes less than $11,000, well below the poverty line. So, if these children come to term, they will end up growing up in difficult circumstances and making the job of getting out of poverty more difficult for those who will raise them.

Pro-choice advocates worry about the inevitable "backstreet abortion" if abortion is made illegal, and they also worry about the quality of women's lives if they are denied the basic autonomy of reproductive self-control. The pro-life theorist, on the other hand, will see the social problem as just another manifestation of the rampant immorality of the modern age. The pro-life theorist will argue that it is quite possible to grow up "decent" in a poor household, and that to believe otherwise is to be elitist. The pro-life advocate considers the element of autonomy in reproduction more of a matter of "convenience" than a lifeplan that has priority over the continued existence of the fetus. It should be clear from this radical disagreement over the value of women's reproductive autonomy that we are dealing with deep-seated moral beliefs. The one side believes that self-realization through the development of one's lifeplan (one's "biographical life") is all important, while the pro-life theorist points to the sanctity of human "biological life." This radical disagreement over basic beliefs makes it possible to understand the violent emotions that have been unleashed in the political battle over abortion.

POLITICAL TACTICS: CIVIL DISOBEDIENCE AT THE CLINIC

In March of 1993, Michael Griffin shot and killed Dr. David Gunn, an abortion doctor outside an abortion clinic in Pensacola, Florida. This most extreme of actions shocked the nation as well as activists on both sides of the issue but was hardly unexpected, given the intensity of the abortion debate. With the ever-increasing acrimony as well as positions unlikely to change, the stage is set for even more violent action. Whatever one thinks of Michael Griffin, the conclusion he came to is easy enough to understand: If one is completely certain that the fetus is a person, and if millions of these people are being killed, it takes only utilitarian reasoning to arrive at the conclusion that killing one person to save hundreds is morally defensible. A proponent of this form of reasoning is Randall Terry, the leader of Operation Rescue, a militant anti-abortion group. Upon hearing what Griffin had done he remarked, "We will not be outraged over the one death and not the other 4000 precious human beings killed today by abortion."[5]

Most people find an obvious contradiction in Griffin's actions. Killing someone because they have killed also implicates oneself. We must also remember that utilitarian reasoning is not open to Griffin, since the basis for his action was a Biblical commandment. When *Time* magazine entitled its story "Thou Shalt Not Kill," the editors clearly meant to elicit our sense of contradiction.[5] The Biblical commandment is unambiguous; there are no exceptions for a greater good.

Although the pro-choice camp has as yet refrained from violent action to protect the right of choice, it is not hard to imagine that such a response could be forthcoming as the other side grows increasingly violent. Clearly, what is needed is a plea for tolerance and a deeper understanding of why attitudes toward abortion lead to such emotional disagreement.

The lengths to which people will go for the sake of their beliefs differ:

1. Some hold the pro-life or pro-choice position but don't work to bring it about.
2. Some work toward laws for or against abortion.
3. Some are willing to engage in peaceful protest.
4. Some are willing to engage in violence to change behavior or beliefs.
5. Some believe that murder or terror is an appropriate response to certain political problems.

Short of totally eliminating them, there have also been attempts by pro-life forces to reduce the number of abortions. The Hyde Amendment of 1980 cut off government funding for Medicaid abortions. The reasoning was that since pro-life people pay taxes they should have the right to restrict the spending of their tax money to moral purposes. There is also what has been called "the gag rule." Until Clinton became president and eliminated it, doctors were not allowed to offer abortion as an alternative to pregnant women. We are likely to see laws coming into and out of effect as pro-choice and pro-life politicians come into and out of office.

TRADITIONALISM VS. MODERNISM

The abortion issue is just the most obvious point of conflict between people with different world views. There have been studies of the social backgrounds of pro-life and pro-choice activists, and the results are revealing. Pro-life activists tend to be more traditional and religious. They believe that sex should be reserved for marriage, if not merely for procreation. Pro-choice activists tend to be less traditional and religious, more career oriented with higher incomes. They also tend to believe that sex is a natural expression of oneself. What is clear is that we have the well-known conflict between conservative traditionalists and liberal modernists. The former are distrustful of deviations from tradition and see society's problems as the result of straying from the traditional mores. Pro-choice activists, on the other hand, see the social problems as a result of traditionalists failing to realize the changing of the times. They argue that it is precisely the traditionalist rejection of sex education and contraception that is the source of the problem. In the modernists' view, there would be many fewer abortions if these reforms were allowed to be instituted without resistance. For traditionalists, it is only their own resistance to the full implementation of the liberal program that prevents wholesale chaos and immorality. But since we are already in a "chaotic" situation, pro-life advocates are relying rather heavily on the possibility of a religious revival that many would resist.

Another point of view of the Traditionalism/Modernism perspective on abortion is possible. Some would argue that the pro-life position is actually the more progressive of the two. The argument tries to place the attempt to give rights to the fetus within the line of development we have seen in the civil rights and women's movements. Just as people realized that African Americans and women deserve the same rights as white males, now, it is argued, we must extend the liberalizing program to the fetus.

ABORTION AND THE FREEDOM OF RELIGION

Given that the abortion disagreement lies so deeply in our religious and moral frameworks, one is led to ask whether abortion should be regarded as a case of religious disagreement and therefore subject to the constitutional guarantee of freedom of religion. If one's view of abortion is really a result of one's religious beliefs, it would seem that the government should play no role in restricting it. It should come as no surprise that pro-life theorists reject the idea that their views on abortion are the result of their religious views but rather maintain that they are the result of basic moral reasoning. They point to the fact that, while the above characterization of pro-choice and pro-life activists is true, it is also true that many nonreligious people and members of the more liberal religious sects are also opposed to abortion. They also point out that freedom of religion is not absolute. One cannot murder or steal and then argue that it should be allowed because it is part of his or her religion. Since the issue is whether abortion is murder, the freedom of religion does not come into play.

Pro-choice theorists argue that even if disagreement on abortion cuts across the various religions, as well as atheism, it is still the case that the issue is one that lies rather deep, as deep as any religious views one might have. Remember, abortion views tend to reflect one's most deeply held beliefs, so even if the views are not religious in the partisan sense, they are equally profound. It is argued that the disagreement is so profound that the best solution would be the same one that resulted from the religious wars of earlier centuries: tolerance.

Many people see tolerance as the best way out of our present situation. It is unlikely that one side is going to come up with an argument that will cause the opponents to suddenly "see the light" and switch sides. One problem with this continuing controversy over abortion is the way that it skews politics. People are more and more becoming one-issue voters rather than assessing the candidates' positions on all of the issues. We may also be losing good candidates because they live in areas in which the majority has a different view on the abortion issue. On the other hand, some argue that one's abortion stance is crucial to determining whether or not a politician understands the changing needs of women and modern social conditions generally (pro-choice) or the decline in moral standards (pro-life).

THE ENVIRONMENTAL PERSPECTIVE

Recall Thomson's carpet-seed children, whereby we tried to imagine children being the result of airborne seeds. Such a possibility is certainly far-fetched, but it does bring up an important point, namely that it is a contingent result of the evolutionary process that we have as many children as we do. One can easily imagine humans reproducing like frogs and many other creatures and giving birth to thousands of offspring in order to survive as a species in a situation of high infant mortality. One can also imagine that, as humans advanced, they could eventually overcome the environmental forces that make it necessary to have so many offspring. Imagine that the only way to prevent our froglike humans from developing into adults is abortion. In such a case not only would it be permissible to have abortions, it would probably be necessary since the world would otherwise be quickly overpopulated. It would be necessary, also, if we were to have anything like the family structure that we have now. The suggestion is that human life, at least in its early stages, is not as valuable as some make it out to be. What would turn out to be more important would be a strong family structure. Once a family was ready to commit to a child, the sanctity of life would come into play, but fetuses would have very little value without such commitment. This is in line with an environmental perspective that sees humans as members of a biotic community with duties to maintain a balance of numbers with other members of that community. One cannot derive a right to abortion directly from the need to curb population growth—contraception is better for a number of reasons—but an aggressive attitude toward family planning fits well with an attitude of respect for nature.

THE FAMILY PLANNING PERSPECTIVE

The family planning perspective also asks why we should favor accidental babies over planned babies. What gives a baby who happens to be conceived when a woman is the age of 18 more right to life than the one she would have had at 28? Given that people have the right to choose the size of their family—something that will be necessary in the long run anyway—it makes sense that they should also have the right to choose at what point they will have their children. Optimally, people want children to come when the family is financially and emotionally stable. Marriage is difficult enough without the added strain of unwanted children. Given the social problems of poverty, single parenthood, child abuse, and so on, some argue that it may be time to reconsider what is really important to the family structure.

A pro-life perspective would regard such a point of view as absurd and maybe even horrifying. Once a baby is conceived it is a person in their view, thus possessing a right to life. In such a frame of reference, it makes no sense to compare this baby with a possible baby ten years from now. Rights only belong to existing beings. The pro-life view would see family planning as another example of the decadent culture of permissiveness.

SUMMARY

Abortion is an extremely emotional issue in that it makes us consider some very important and deep moral concepts, such as personhood and the value of human life. While it is important to understand the facts of fetal development, there is no getting around the problem of philosophical disagreement over fundamentals. Nor can we ignore important social realities such as the liberation of women and the problem of teenage mothers. Abortion also requires that we review our moral intuitions. We discussed various analogies in order to determine whether our intuitions can yield a consistent moral position on abortion.

Whatever your view on abortion, it should be clear that the issue is a difficult one that reaches to the depths of our most profound thoughts on what is important in life. Nothing indicates that the controversy will end anytime soon, so how is a sensitive person to regard her opponents on the issue? If one imagines that a fetus is a baby, how much effort on its behalf is rational? An adult who rushes into the street to save a toddler who has entered the pathway of an onrushing car would be considered a hero. What, then, is so extraordinary about blocking a doorway or lying down in front of an abortion clinic, if what you see yourself doing is saving babies? If, on the other hand, your view of a fetus is that of a piece of tissue—even one with remarkable potential, but still only a piece of tissue—jumping in front of cars or blocking doorways is very strange behavior indeed.

Perhaps what is missing in the debate is a level of tolerance and civility that considers the opposing view to be wrong but perhaps rational. Following the tragic killing of Dr. Gunn, the pro-choice advocates began to call the pro-life advocates "terrorists" while the pro-life movement continued to cast the pro-choice side as "baby killers." It is not likely that "baby killers" and "terrorists" are the kinds of people who will be able to sit down and reason together. Confrontations have become increasingly violent and costly as one town after another becomes a battleground.

Is there a possibility that one day people on both sides of the issue will be able to set aside their differences and come to some agreement? Maybe there is some hope in the fact that the authors of this book disagree on the abortion issue yet were able to work together in order to write this book.

CLARIFICATION EXERCISES

A. On March 28, 1992, the *Wall Street Journal* reported that the New Jersey Supreme Court had tossed out the appeal of a man seeking to stop his girlfriend from having an abortion. Much has been written about the woman's right over her body, but relatively little about the father's rights. Does a man have the right to veto an abortion? Does he have the right to veto a pregnancy? What duties logically follow from such rights?

Use this exercise to assess the doctrine that says that for every right you have there must be someone with a correlative duty.

B. Since 1988, RU 486, or mifepristone, has been used by 80,000 women in France for early first-trimester abortions. RU 486 has been found effective and safe in 96% of abortions in

a French study. What is the appropriate position to take on RU 486, "the abortion pill"?
RU 486 is a drug that prevents the blastocyst (the zygote) from embedding in the uterine wall. It does this by blocking the naturally produced hormone, progesterone, the absence of which causes the uterine wall to shed its lining and any fertilized egg.

The Ethics of RU 486: Is the zygote a person? Review the criteria of personhood proposed by Warren to make your decision.

The Politics of RU 486: RU 486 is made by a French Pharmaceutical Company, Roussel-Uclaf, that also makes other products. Pro-life activists have threatened to boycott the company's other products if it markets the pill in the United States. Is this an appropriate action for a pro-life activist to take? What if the pill turns out to have other important medical uses?

How is RU 486 different from the IUD? The cervical cap? The traditional pill? Compare the different forms of contraception with regard to the abortion issue.

C. A recent development in contraceptive technology is the "underarm pill" called **Norplant.** It is a low-dosage, slow-release pill implanted under the arm that lasts for five years.

We have discussed the severe problems of teen pregnancy in some areas. How would you feel about mandatory implantation in teenage girls in problem areas for example, (high schools where 90 percent of all girls are pregnant before graduation)?

What about a national policy of RU 486 implantation? Should we implant all girls of a certain age to avoid discrimination? We could respect the wishes of certain groups who would reject the implantation, so one could also petition not to receive the pill. But then should the state be required to help to raise a child who is the result?

Should the parents who engage in child abuse be required to wear an underarm pill?

D. Some abortion foes object to fetal tissue research on the grounds that it will lead to more abortions, or at least to a feeling that the immorality of abortion may be partially offset by the fact that the tissue will be put to good use. Is this fear justified?

E. Michigan has a parental consent law stating that minors must get permission from parents or a judge before having an abortion. Imagine a similar law that adds a provision that if the parent refuses to allow the abortion it is the parent's responsibility to raise the child, not the minor's. Which would be the better law?

F. Rule utilitarians regard rights as human creations, as merely good rules that yield the greatest happiness for the greatest number. Consider the right to life from the perspective of the rule utilitarian and determine whether such a view could support the pro-life side, the pro-choice side, or both.

G. Some states have passed what is called the "informed consent" law. Such a law would require anyone considering an abortion to wait 24 hours and to view pictures of fetuses at the same stage as her fetus. Would such a law be a good idea? Do we require heart patients to witness open-heart surgery before they undergo the operation themselves? Is this a good analogy?

H. Do health professionals have the duty to participate in abortions even if they find them morally repugnant?

I. Examine the following statistics: What, if anything, can we learn from them? Which side does each statistic support?[6]
   1. In 1989, there were 1,396,658 abortions reported.
   2. In the same year, there were 346 abortions per 1,000 live births.
   3. 80 percent of all abortions are performed on unmarried women.
   4. .01 percent of all abortions take place after 24 weeks.
   5. 50 percent of all pregnancies are unintended.
   6. 57 percent of all teenage pregnacies in 1989 were terminated by abortion.
   7. 1 percent of all women having abortions have been informed the fetus has a defect.

8. 55 percent of all teenagers who have an abortion inform their parents.

9. Childbirth is eleven times more dangerous than abortion.

10. 16,000 women seek abortions each year as a result of rape or incest.

11. 2,000 copies of self-abortion videos have been sold to women's groups since 1989.

12. 500,000 women die each year from pregnancy-related problems.

Use these statistics to examine the relationship between facts and values.

REFERENCES AND SUGGESTED READING

1. Mary Anne Warren, "On the Moral and Legal Status of Abortion," in *The Problem of Abortion,* ed. Joel Feinberg (Belmont, CA: Wadsworth Books, 1984).

2. Mary Anne Warren, "On the Moral and Legal Status of Abortion."

3. Michael Tooley, "A Defense of Abortion and Infanticide," in *The Problem of Abortion,* ed. Joel Feinberg (Belmont, CA: Wadsworth Books, 1984).

4. Judith Thomson, "A Defense of Abortion," in *The Problem of Abortion,* ed. Joel Feinberg (Belmont, CA: Wadsworth Books, 1984).

5. "Thou Shalt Not Kill," *Time,* 22 March 1993.

6. "One Doctor Down, How Many More?" *Time,* 22 March 1993.

7. *The Detroit Free Press,* 18 February 1992.

CHAPTER 10

Ethical Issues and Genetic Science

INSTRUCTIONAL GOAL

Upon completion of this chapter the reader should understand the various areas of genetic research and the moral problems that are associated with them.

INSTRUCTIONAL OBJECTIVES

By the end of the chapter the reader should be able to:

1. Understand the purpose, practice, benefits, and dangers of genetic screening.
2. Understand the benefits of prenatal genetic testing and how it leads to the moral issues that surround abortion.
3. Describe the dangers of utilizing genetic research for the purpose of eugenics.
4. Explain the promise of the human genome project.
5. Understand the scientific advances possible with recombinant DNA as well as the dangers that unregulated research can create.
6. Put all the issues that are raised in this chapter in the context of the Faust legend.
7. Explain how ethical problems with genetics make necessary a new virtue of family planning with guidelines that help us utilize genetic counseling in an ethical manner.
8. Explain the promise of gene therapy.

Glossary

Allele: A variant form of a given gene, which may determine a trait such as having type-O or type-A blood.

Cystic Fibrosis: A disease that causes the accumulation of mucus in the lungs and clogs small passages. The disease is fatal.

148

Dominant Gene: A gene that only needs to be present in one parent in order to have a 50–50 chance of affecting each child.

Down Syndrome: A condition in which a person is born with an extra chromosome (47), which leads to varying degrees of retardation, a shorter lifespan, and other ailments.

Eugenics: The practice of breeding humans in order to produce superior offspring.

Gene Marker: A visible or detectable trait that is inherited along with an unknown gene.

Genetic Carriers: A person who carries a defective gene that, when combined in reproduction with a similar one from another person, may yield a genetic defect. A carrier does exhibit symptoms of the disease.

Genetic Disease: A disease caused by a genetic abnormality.

Genetic Predisposition to Disease: A genetically determined susceptibility to certain health problems. It does not cause the disease itself, but, in combination with behavioral and environmental factors, can increase a person's chances of getting a certain disease.

Genetic Screening: The practice of inspecting the genetic makeup of parents for abnormalities.

Gene Therapy: The treatment of genetic diseases by the administration of genes to correct an absent or defective gene.

Genome: The complete genetic makeup of a species.

Heterozygous: Children inherit one allele from each parent. When the child has one, say, for Sickle Cell Anemia, and one that is normal, we say the child is heterozygous.

Homozygous: When a child possesses two identical alleles (one from each parent) for a variant gene, we say the child is homozygous.

Huntington's Disease: A disease that strikes in middle age, initially causing clumsiness and eventually a complete loss of control, both mental and physical. The condition is caused by a degeneration of the brain, particularly the part that controls movement, mood, and thought.

Monogenic: A disease caused by a single gene.

Polygenic: A disease caused by a combination of genes.

Recessive Gene: A gene that must be present in both parents for a child to inherit the gene. On average, when both parents are carriers, the child will have a 1-in-4 chance of inheriting the disease and a 50-50 chance of becoming a carrier. There is also a 1-in-4 chance of being free of the gene altogether.

Recombinant DNA: The practice of altering DNA by splicing parts of one into another.

Sickle Cell: A disease in which the red blood cells fail to provide the muscles with enough oxygen, thus causing excruciating muscle cramps and damage to organs when the sickled cells clog the small blood vessels.

It is clear that the enormous increase in the power of the doctor raises many questions which have never previously been raised—"Science has made us gods before we are even worthy of being men"[1]

Ethics in Medical Progress

One day a woman's father comes home and starts ranting and raving. She has never quite seen him like this. His limbs begin moving in strange ways, and later, he begins to have seizures. Finally, the doctors have the diagnosis: **Huntington's disease.** Now she finds out that, because her father's disease is the result of a dominant gene, she has a 50–50 chance of getting it herself. This is the story of Frances.[2] It is not a happy story, but it is true, and it is repeated all too often. There is no cure for Huntington's disease, and it develops between a person's 30s and 50s, so one often finds out only after having passed the disease to one's own children. If the damage has been done, is it better not to know? After all, fifty years is a lifetime, even if it does not match our average life expectancy. Still, there is great hope, for researchers have moved fast in first finding a **marker** for the gene that causes Huntington's disease, and now in finding the actual gene that causes it.[3] However, the great hope that we have is associated with potential danger, for knowledge is power, and the knowledge gained in finding the Huntington's gene is the same as that used in bioengineering—potentially one of the greatest but also most dangerous developments of human intelligence. But the stakes are high. Twenty percent of the 250,000 birth defects in children are due to known genetic causes. Should we just let **genetic disease** continue if we have the power to stop it or at least lessen its impact? The consensus so far seems to be that we should move forward, but we should be clear regarding what it means to move forward in this area.

> After thousands of years of engineering the cold remains of the earth into utilities, human beings are now setting out to engineer the internal biology of living organisms . . . The transition is indeed staggering.[4]

MEDICAL PROGRESS: A FAUSTIAN BARGAIN?

Modern science has achieved more than we could have dreamed possible. There is no denying the good that science has done for us. On the other hand, there is no doubt that the dangers are just as great as the benefits we have gained. Can we go too far in our attempts to understand nature? Have we gone beyond the limits of human responsibility? These are questions that arise when we consider current research in genetics and attempts to use this knowledge for the improvement of human life. Genes are the basic carriers of the information that makes us what we are. If we reach the point at which we understand these biological building blocks, will the power that comes with such knowledge be too much for humanity to use responsibly? These same questions were raised with the development of atomic science and have yet to be adequately resolved. For example, antinuclear activists argue that the consequences of a nuclear accident at a power plant outweigh the possible benefits of the plants in operation, and that the problems with waste disposal have yet to be overcome. Such questions are arising more and more in all areas of science, but genetic science has possibly the greatest potential for good and ill. In this chapter, we will examine recent developments in genetic science, particularly as it applies to medicine, and attempt to determine how we should negotiate our way through the forest of ethical issues that arise when we seek to understand and employ our understanding.

There are several areas of genetic inquiry that raise ethical questions. In our attempt to understand the causes of and develop treatments for genetically caused disease, we are naturally led to employ our knowledge for human benefit. Two areas of research are testing potential parents and prenatal testing of unborn children. Moreover, the ethical questions that arise concern the actions to be taken once the test results are in hand. Are we to prevent a couple from having children if they are likely to give birth to a genetically diseased infant? Should parents be allowed to, or even forced to, abort genetically diseased fetuses? These are difficult questions, and there are no easy answers. Nevertheless, we must come to terms with them because the future is now; we have the ability to engage in such testing.

GENETICS AS SOCIAL POLICY

Other ethical issues arise when we consider the possibility of turning genetic testing into social policy. Some suggest that all parents be tested for genetic diseases in order to avoid the social and personal costs of genetic impairment. Others worry that this will lead to a coercive policy of abortion or of preventing parents from having children. Such policies raise still further issues when they are directed to certain ends, as they are with eugenics. **Eugenics** is the practice of manipulating the genes of offspring through either breeding or genetic alteration. Should we attempt to eliminate some or all genetic abnormalities? Should we attempt to improve the race of human beings by increasing intelligence through genetic selection?

But scientists are not only involved with genetic testing; they are also engaged in an enterprise called "the human genome project." The task is to "map" the 100,000 genes that make up the 46 human chromosomes, which altogether comprise the "human genome." The **genome** is the blueprint contained in each cell that guides the development of the human being. The ethical worries regarding this issue are more vague; they have as much to do with the idea of humans possessing such "God-like" knowledge as they have to do with the application of the knowledge. From certain theological points of view, the mere possession of such profound knowledge is immoral; only God should have such knowledge. The idea is that the attempt to gain such knowledge is hubris or excessive pride. It is suggested that we leave such knowledge to God and concern ourselves with more mundane tasks.

GENETIC ENGINEERING

The recombinant DNA process is the most dramatic technological tool to date in the growing biotechnological arsenal. The biologist is learning how to manipulate, recombine and reorganize living tissue into new forms and shapes, just as his craftsmen

ancestors did by firing inanimate matter. The speed of the discoveries is truly phenome-
nal. It is estimated that biological knowledge is currently doubling every five years, and
in the field of genetics . . . We are virtually hurling ourselves into the age of bio-
technology.[4]

Research into Recombinant DNA is indeed a marvel of modern science, but it also
brings forth some of the greatest fears of all. Scientists are now genetically altering
organisms for various purposes. We have recently heard about genetically altered
fruits and vegetables, but the range of experiments is extremely varied. (A recent
development has been to grow plastic potatoes!) The fear is that experimenters will
develop organisms that will endanger humans or other living beings. The possibilities are the stuff of science fiction, and such fears have led to calls for restricting
this research or even banning it altogether. Such calls have decreased in recent years,
but they have not been completely silenced. Additional issues have arisen concerning conflict of interest among scientists who are supported by government but who
turn to the marketplace for additional compensation.[5] The ethical issues that arise
involve those listed above in connection with the human genome project, but others
worry whether scientists can be trusted with the awesome responsibilities that come
with such dangerous research. Can we rely on scientists to take the necessary
precautions to keep the organisms they create harmless to human beings? In what
follows, we will explore these issues in greater detail.

GENETIC TESTING

The Promise and Peril of Genetic Testing: Doctors can test couples to see if it is
possible that they will give birth to a genetically impaired infant. For example, we
can now test couples for **sickle cell,** a disease that deforms red blood cells into thin,
elongated sickle-shaped forms and causes anemia, cough, and muscle cramps. Sickle
cell occurs only when both parents are carriers of the recessive gene. If both parents
are carriers, there is a 25 percent chance that the child will have the disease. Is this too
much of a risk for parents to take? Depending upon how paternalistic we are, we
might either (1) not allow them to have children, (2) suggest strongly that they do
not have children, (3) refuse to pay the medical expenses (this would be a decision
for insurance companies and/or government), or (4) merely leave it up to the parents
whether to take the risk. Most would leave the decision up to the parents, but some
would argue that the parents should not be allowed to have a child when the risk is
so high. It is argued that it is unfair to bring a child into the world knowing that it
will have such a heavy burden to bear.

Sickle cell is instructive, however, in that it is a disease that primarily afflicts
people of African descent. To refuse to allow people children who are members of a
minority may suggest racist motives. But there are other diseases that are not so
selective; are we to restrict people afflicted with nonracially connected genetic
disease? Many people believe that it is their right to bear children, however they turn
out. It is further argued that there are many afflictions that are not genetically caused

or cannot be tested for; why might such people be allowed to be born but not those with a disposition to diseases we can test for? The assumption here is that existence is a good thing; for some it may not be, and then testing would be preventing injury. This raises a deep problem: Can existence be an injury?

At first glance, human existence could be understood as an injury in utilitarian terms if the prospective life would likely contain more unhappiness than happiness. But this will not do, because ordinary life is a veil of tears for many people. To be useful for our purposes in the argument that asserts that existence can be an injury, it must be the case that bodily or mental impairment must be significantly greater than that which most people must face. This is certainly true for many diseases, and this would provide us with grounds to argue that existence can be an injury; therefore it would be immoral for such a person to be brought into the world.

Some argue that the perspective employed in such an argument is not the correct one. The proper perspective is that of the person afflicted, and from such a perspective any sort of existence may be preferable to none at all. It may be that great suffering may be endurable if just a little happiness is possible, and this is almost always the case. There is also the problem of anticipating what a future person would prefer. Given the difficulties of such calculations, some argue that there can be no good argument against having children.

A middle ground may be found by referring to actual cases. Some diseases offer only a brief and painful existence, while others are so seriously painful and prolonged that the question of a worthwhile life is out of the question. On the other hand, some diseases are not as severe. Take, for example, **Down syndrome.** Such children are afflicted with serious problems, but the severity varies widely. It is often pointed out that Down syndrome children frequently lead happy lives.

Some argue that we must also never underestimate the human spirit and its ability to overcome adversity. As a notable example, Helen Keller is known for having overcome devastating odds to lead a fulfilling life. The response to this argument is that one case does not a policy make. We must ground any moral policy in the reality of the overwhelming majority of cases. Policy should aim at the majority, and exceptions to the rule—the hard cases—should be regarded as exceptional. It may be too much to expect that all those with Helen Keller's afflictions be able to achieve what she did.

We may be able to test for **genetic predispositions** in the future. Some people are more genetically predisposed to certain diseases (such as cancer) and to react to toxic chemicals that cause diseases. Roughly 10 percent of the population have bodies that produce enzymes that combine with hydrocarbons and produce carcinogenic substances. One can imagine companies refusing to hire potential employees who are genetically disposed to diseases caused by the toxic chemicals used in certain industries. In fact, this is already happening without the benefit of genetic testing; the mere occurrence of several instances of a disease in a family has led companies to gauge the cost and availability of insurance accordingly. One can, therefore, assume that as actual tests become available the possibilities for discrimination will be great. Given that we have no control over our genetic make-up, the fairness of such practices must be questioned.

PRENATAL TESTING

Prenatal testing brings up additional difficulties. It is sometimes possible to test for genetic abnormalities after conception but not before. There are three types of prenatal testing: amniocentesis, chorionic villus sampling, and viewing the fetus with either ultrasound, radiography, or fiber optics. Amniocentesis is a procedure in which amniotic fluid is removed and analyzed for evidence of defects. Amniocentesis is generally performed after the fourteenth week and the risk to the woman and fetus are relatively small. Chorionic villus sampling takes cells directly from the fetus and can be employed up to six weeks earlier and is just as safe as amniocentesis. However, both procedures have risks, so they are not generally employed unless the doctor has reason to believe the fetus may have some genetic or developmental disorder. Viewing the fetus can be done early in the pregnancy, but it only reveals defects that can be determined through visual inspection of an image of the fetus. If a defect is detected, the only alternative (at this time) to bringing the fetus to term would be abortion, with the attendant difficulties of that issue. Those opposed to abortion may be opposed to prenatal testing, since it may lead to abortion. And if it doesn't lead to abortion, such testing only increases the unhappiness associated with defective newborns by letting the parents know sooner. Those unopposed to abortion may consider it their right to have their unborn fetuses tested for genetic abnormalities, so that they could abort in the early stages of the pregnancy.

THE ROLE OF PARENTS

Virtue ethics gives us a special perspective on this question. It is the role of parents to make many decisions for their children, including the decision of life and death (or nonexistence) prior to conception and birth (assuming one is pro-abortion). One can construct a virtue ethics position that puts the decision completely in the hands of the parents. Thus, if a couple wishes to take on the burden of raising a defective child, it is morally acceptable. It must also be added that having such a child would entail duties that would go beyond those that parents of normal children would be required to assume. (Society may also gain a voice in the decision if the cost of raising the child is carried by society to any great extent. Is it legitimate knowingly to bring a child into the world with serious defects when one also knows that one cannot pay the expenses?) Prior commitments to society must be made if one takes on a risk knowing that society may very well have to carry part or all of the economic burden of tending to a child's health. But this perspective also puts the decision not to have children (or to abort) completely in the hands of parents. This would mean that parents would have the right to abort a child with characteristics that many would consider acceptable. Take, for example, the case of the Down's syndrome child previously mentioned. A couple may have a wish for a child who can share in their preference for a rather intellectual existence, an existence that is out of the question for any Down syndrome child.

Many would accept the virtue ethics perspective when it indicates that parents may bring a defective child into the world if they wish but they would not accept the alternative side of the equation that permits parents to abort children deemed unacceptable to them for less than extremely serious reasons. Clearly, one's position on the abortion issue and the concept of personhood come into play. If one is inclined to accept abortion, then both sides of the virtue ethics perspective make sense. If one does not accept abortion as a morally acceptable practice, then one would argue that it would be acceptable to refrain from conceiving such children but that it would not be acceptable to abort such a child once conceived.

THE POLITICS OF SCREENING

Testing large populations (screening) has a checkered history. The early sickle-cell anemia screening laws are instructive.[6] The science of testing got caught up in a whirlwind of well-intentioned legislation in the early stages of the civil rights movement. It was a way of doing good for African Americans, a group of people who were becoming increasingly important. But alas, legislators are not scientists. The early legislation was often poorly written and sometimes directed at the wrong target populations.

One consistent mistake was to refer to carriers of the sickle cell as diseased. To have the disease one must have inherited the allele from both parents, whereas carriers have only inherited the allele from one parent. An unanticipated problem came up as paternity discrepancies arose. If a child turned out to be **heterozygous** and neither parent was heterozygous, then it became clear that someone else was involved in the reproductive process. There are many instances where this sort of revelation has led to the breakup of otherwise stable families.[7]

Other mistakes occurred. The state of Virginia, for example, mandated that all convicts be tested for the disease, when inmates generally have few immediate plans for reproduction. Some states used testing methods that were not the most accurate available and thus achieved an unacceptably high number of incorrect positive results. Finally, there is the issue of confidentiality. Few states were prepared to protect the confidentiality of the patients. It was feared that discrimination in employment and insurance would result, or at the least that a social stigma would be attached to those identified as carriers. The lesson of the sickle cell experience shows us that genetic screening requires wisdom, sensitivity, and most important, good science. We must not allow well-intentioned proposals to become practice without paying close attention to the procedures and the consequences.

EUGENICS

> The children of the good parents they will take to a rearing pen in the care of nurses living apart in a certain section of the city; the children of inferior parents, or any child of the others born defective, they will hide, as is fitting, in a secret and unknown place. Plato, *The Republic,* Book V, 460C (380 B.C.).[8]

It is clear that Plato is referring to the practice of infanticide for diseased or disabled newborns. It is also clear that this practice is conceived to be part of a more general practice of **eugenics,** for Plato goes on to say "if the breed of guardians is to remain pure." Sometimes what we think to be new choices are really quite old. After all, stock breeding is a form of eugenics. The dairy cow of today is a far cry from the wild cow from which it is descended. Our most recent experience with eugenics came when the Nazi experiments on human beings were revealed. It is, therefore, understandable if people are a bit apprehensive over any renaissance of eugenic ideas. Nevertheless, we should always give proposals a hearing lest some suspect that we are avoiding discussion out of fear of the truth.

The ability to screen and prenatally test for genetic disease raises the possibility that we could eliminate genetic diseases with a policy of negative eugenics or even improve the genetic pool of humanity by selecting for positive attributes, positive eugenics. A moderate policy of eugenics that has the intention of eliminating the most serious genetic diseases seems sensible enough, but even such a moderate approach is fraught with difficulties. The number of people carrying a recessive gene is rather large, and it is difficult to justify preventing such people from reproducing merely because they have a recessive gene. Given that it is impossible to have a genetically impaired infant with only one parent contributing a recessive gene for, say, sickle-cell anemia, it would be hard to justify preventing such a couple from having children. On the other hand, if we do not eliminate these recessive genes, we will never overcome genetic disease.

An extreme program of negative eugenics faces practical difficulties that make it almost, if not in fact, impossible to implement. Could we eliminate all genetic disease? Since the majority of people carry at least one recessive gene for some genetic disease, a radical policy of negative eugenics would eliminate a large portion of the human population. But there is a more important question to ask: Would we want to eliminate all genetic disease? There are dangers involved in shrinking the gene pool. Our resistance to various sorts of biological attack is dependent to a great degree on our genetic variety. Take, for example, sickle-cell anemia. We know the disease only from its negative effects here in the United States, but in malarial Africa, where the disease developed, being a carrier of the disease functions to ward off the effects of malaria.

A program of positive eugenics—here understood to include not only breeding but genetic intervention—attempts to improve the gene pool by increasing the numbers of those with positive attributes. A 1992 Harris Poll has shown that, if this technology were available, many parents would make use of it. It is unlikely that we could ever develop anything like a "superhuman," but parents may be able to specify specific traits they would prefer to hand down to their children. There would be pressure upon parents (and the same would be true of nations) to utilize positive eugenics in order to increase their children's chances in a competitive market. But the problem ultimately is a scientific one; it is almost impossible to imagine a successful scientific program of eugenics, positive or negative. At this stage, the conclusion seems to be that our best course of action is to use genetic testing to help individuals rather than to alter the genetic makeup of humanity.

THE HUMAN GENOME PROJECT

As previously indicated, the human genome project is the attempt to map the whole human genome, the complete genetic makeup of the human being. Given that this is pure research, the only question to ask is whether such knowledge is proper for humans to possess. Critics of the human genome project could point to the character of Faust (or Dr. Faustus) in order to show how one can be led astray by the unquenchable thirst for knowledge. Dr. Faustus is a scholar so determined to possess more and more knowledge—especially concerning the deepest subjects such as the secret of life and afterlife—that he is willing to trade his soul to the devil for it. Faust makes the bargain and is happy with the bargain until the devil comes for his payment. In the same way, we will be happy with what our knowledge will bring us, but we will be devastated when we are called upon to pay the fee. Like Icarus, we will fly too high, and our wings will melt. This is, in fact, how Marlowe understood the character of Dr. Faustus.

> Till swoll'n with cunning, of a self-conceit,
> His waxen wings did mount above his reach
> And melting, heavens conspired his overthrow![9]

The point of the Faust and Icarus stories is generally that humankind should recognize its limitations; the failure to do so is to commit the sin of excessive pride or hubris. In secular terms, we say that humankind is in danger of overreaching its proper boundaries.

The key worry behind overreaching is that there is inevitably some disaster that comes as a result. The question is whether there will be any such fee, for no one has made any pacts with the devil in setting up the human genome project.

Some argue that there are no limits to human knowledge and that there shouldn't be. Such fears, it could be argued, are the result of theological beliefs that are no longer held. The theological basis for the Faustian view is that humans have a predetermined place in the scheme of things, and to move beyond this predetermined place is sacrilegious. Religious people do tend to believe that humankind has a place in God's plan, but most are not terribly sure that the quest for knowledge interferes with that plan; indeed, one can easily imagine that our place is to seek knowledge as a way of better knowing God's plan. For those who are not religious at all, there is no problem with God's plans in the first place. Environmentalists sometimes think of humankind as occupying a certain place in the natural order, but doing so is quite consistent with an unending quest for knowledge. There are dangers, to be sure, but they arise only when knowledge is applied. A discussion of this danger is best left until the next section, on recombinant DNA.

There is a worry on the other side of the question—worry that we will put up artificial barriers to our knowledge and stop short of great discoveries that will radically increase the quality of life. Imagine if we had refrained from discovering the causes of various diseases that we have learned to cure or prevent. The fear is that we would be doing something similar if we stopped now in our quest for knowledge. Fears of the improper extension of human knowledge therefore seem to be unfounded unless one believes that the application of knowledge inevitably follows its acquisition. The question ultimately comes down to whether mankind can be trusted to use (or not use) the knowledge in question.

RECOMBINANT DNA RESEARCH

A recent issue of *Time* reported the following story:

> **Plastic Plants**
> Taking a cue from Rumpelstilskin, who spun straw into gold, botanists managed to coax a lowly potted plant into producing plastic. Using genetic-engineering techniques, researchers redirected the plant's starch-storing apparatus into making PHB, a plastic that is biodegradable.[10]

The application of the knowledge gained from the human genome project is likely to be in the field of **recombinant DNA.** Scientists recombine the genetic material from one organism to another for various reasons. Sometimes it is done to improve a plant in some way, for example, to make it less susceptible to spoilage and damage, to ripen it sooner, and so on. Scientists also recombine DNA to create organisms that will attack pests of one sort or another. There have been attempts to create an organism that eats oil, for use in dealing with oil slicks. And, of course, the future holds the prospect of genetic intervention in human beings, either to combat disease or to eliminate a propensity for disease. The possibilities are endless.

Our experiences with nuclear physics give many cause for concern, and the fears associated with genetic research are similar. One fear is that such knowledge will be used by the military as another way to kill people, with disastrous results for both victim and victor. If a genetically engineered virus or bacteria were used, it would be difficult to contain and could very well attack us as well.

But even the peaceful uses of recombinant DNA technology are worrisome. One never knows if some experimental creature will interact with the natural environment in some negative way. Will we inadvertently create a modern-day Frankenstein? The most commonly used bacteria is E coli, which is found in the stomachs of all human beings. Most creatures created by humans do not do well in the natural environment and are likely to die outside the laboratory, but since the attempts are precisely to create creatures hardy enough to fulfill our purposes in nature the prospect does hold some dangers. Scientists do employ special protocols for dealing with altered genetic materials, so it is unlikely that something will just be flushed down the drain where it can enter the natural environment, but as the technology becomes more common it is likely to be in the hands of people who are not so careful.

The difficult training one must go through to become a genetic scientist will naturally restrict the numbers of those involved, but it is not always the case that people trained in the sciences are also conscious of their ethical duties. There is even one case of a scientist working on an organism to combat a disease affecting trees who was so upset at the delays the regulators were putting him through that he released the organism into the environment on his own. This is the kind of behavior that worries people. Nevertheless, the benefits we may reap from genetic engineering are too great to ignore.

GENETIC PHARMACY

One positive result of genetic engineering has been the development of the "genetic pharmacy." We can now produce substances by genetic alteration that are helpful to many with medical problems. Scientists have modified bacteria to produce human insulin. This is particularly helpful to those diabetics who are allergic to bovine or swine insulin. Vaccines have been produced for hepatitis B and a strain of genital herpes. Genetic pharmacy is one of the most productive and promising applications of genetic engineering.

GENE THERAPY

> It is a profound truth . . . that nature does not know best; that genetic evolution, if we choose to look at it liverishly instead of with fatuous good humor, is a story of waste, makeshift, compromise, and blunder.[11]

Genetic engineering raises the possibility of direct genetic intervention into human beings. Copies of a normal gene are injected into a cell with defective or nonpresent genes. Then the DNA of the cell is induced to incorporate the new gene so that the cell may function properly. If all goes well, when the cell reproduces it passes along the new gene rather than the original. Eventually, the patient acquires a population of good cells that will carry out the proper functions. This method is most likely to be effective when the problem is caused by a single defective gene. Huntington's and sickle cell are this type of disease **(monogenic).** When a disease is the result of a combination of genes **(polygenic),** the potential for genetic treatment is farther off, and most diseases are polygenic. Although gene therapy is extremely difficult, researchers are pushing ahead.

Scientists at the National Institute of Health, for example, are engaged in the attempt to treat cancer patients with gene therapy. Some have argued that we are moving too fast into human experimentation.[12]

The speed at which we proceed is always a problem at the forefront of science and medicine, but the incredible power of gene therapy cautions prudence. We must be very sure that our attempts to improve the hand that nature deals us do not end up making things worse. For example, while the modification of somatic cells (cells that do not affect the genetic make-up of one's children) raises some moral issues, the modification of germ-line cells brings us back to the whole issue of eugenics, with the attendant difficulties. Even short of altering the genetic course of the human race, there are important issues to be raised.

It is likely that we will soon be able to determine the sex of our children. Currently, many parents keep having children until they have one of the sex they prefer. As minor as this consideration is, genetic engineering can help by making sure the first child is a member of the sex preferred by the parents. One obvious problem of giving parents this power is that we may experience an imbalance of males and females. Even now, there are areas of the world where having a female child is regarded negatively, so if the technique of sex determination ever became widely available, problems could result. There is also the question of whether it is right to determine the sex of one's child. What if one chooses the sex, say, male, and the child later learns of the decision? Some might not care. Others might question their whole personality.

THE GENETIC CAUSES OF BEHAVIOR

Another area of potential difficulties arises with the increasing understanding we have of the genetic causes of behavior. Although we are not likely ever to be able to fine-tune the behavior of individuals, even crude genetic modification of behavior could pose risks. One can imagine that some political leaders might prefer passivity for most of their citizenry. Or a political leader might prefer extremely aggressive people to populate the armed forces. Behavior is likely to be polygenic and substantially environmental, so that genetic engineering of this sort is unlikely. Nevertheless, there are some scientists investigating the genetic basis of criminal behavior. Imagine a case in which the presence of a certain gene causes 30 percent of those with the gene to engage in criminal behavior. Also imagine that the other 70 percent turn out to be the leaders of societies. What would be the appropriate action, if any, to take under these circumstances?

CLONING

It is not far-fetched to think that we will eventually be able to clone human beings. Cloning is a process of asexual reproduction in which the nucleus of somatic cells, which contain all of the genetic information necessary to copy an organism, is placed into an egg cell, and an exact copy of the organism will be produced. Plants and even frogs have been successfully cloned. The advantages are easy to imagine. For example, there could always be a ready supply of spare parts in case of injury to the original. One can imagine that being a clone in such circumstances might not be much fun. This is, of course, only a remote possibility, and many believe that analyzing the morality of choices that will be made only in the distant future—if ever—is a useless exercise. On the other hand, waiting until the choice is upon us may not be the wisest course of action either.

SUMMARY

The advances in scientific expertise bring with them moral dilemmas. Genetic research offers great promise; we may soon be able to cure many of the genetically determined diseases and predispositions to disease. We may even be able to improve upon Mother Nature. The question is whether humankind has the wisdom to utilize this knowledge for good without violating moral rules. Only time will tell. Genetic screening will allow parents to know whether their offspring will be afflicted with disease, but in some cases this does nothing more than begin the misery sooner. Prenatal genetic testing will give parents the choice to terminate pregnancies that will lead to defective infants. Genetic testing may also justify discrimination in the minds of many. Eugenics as a state policy is unlikely and will be a long time coming, if ever, but it is fraught with the possibility that charlatans will make such proposals. The human genome project will rank among humankind's greatest achievements once it is completed, and by itself it presents no real moral difficulty; but the application of the knowledge may be more than human wisdom can handle. Recombinant DNA may be the most dangerous as it puts us in the position of creators of whole species that may or may not coexist with humanity and the rest of the natural world. In spite of the dangers, we will proceed, as we should. We may not turn away from the pursuit of knowledge even if some would misuse it.

CLARIFICATION EXERCISES

A. If it became a general practice to abort genetically impaired infants, what would be the likely effect upon genetically impaired infants who are not aborted? Is this a reason to restrict abortions done for this reason?

B. It is likely that we will soon be able not only to detect the sex of the child very early in pregnancy but also to select the sex as well. Assuming such a practice could be done safely, is it morally defensible? What moral difference could it make whether parents have a male or female? Would you want to be able to choose the sex of your children? Would you have wanted your parents to have had this power?

C. There currently are efforts to investigate whether criminal behavior is genetically determined. Aside from the scientific implausibility of all criminal behavior being explained genetically, should someone be discriminated against if his genetic makeup showed him susceptible to such behavior, even prior to that person actually committing a crime?

D. Most work in genetic engineering has been focused on making people better than nature and chance would make them. What would you think of a eugenics policy of producing humans who were inferior to other humans for the purpose of manual labor?

E. Given that the insurance industry is in the business of assessing risks, is it unfair for them to discriminate against individuals if they are found to have a genetic predisposition to, say, mental health problems?

F. Imagine that you have just found out that you have Huntington's disease. You have two children; do you tell them that there is a 50–50 chance that the offspring of someone with Huntington's will have it as well? What if you know that they are not planning to have children? What if they are?

G. Imagine that your parents could have had you genetically altered to be better looking, athletic as a professional athlete, and with genius-level intelligence without altering your basic personality. Would you have preferred that they had done so? If the technology existed, would parents be morally bound to have you genetically altered for the better? What if all the other parents did so except for yours?

H. Can you think of a case where humankind has acquired knowledge without using that knowledge? If not, does that mean we should refrain from continuing the human genome project?

I. Compare the character of Dr. Faustus with the character of Dr. Frankenstein. Does this help us illuminate the dilemmas surrounding genetic engineering?

J. When is the appropriate time to discuss the ethical dilemmas of the future? Do we wait until we are actually faced with the problem, or do we try to anticipate it? Anticipating the problem gives us a longer period of time to try to develop solutions, but it may also be a waste of time if the future does not play out as anticipated. Compare other scientific developments that have led to moral problems, such as atomic science, to recent developments in genetic technology.

K. Would parents be *obligated* to use gene therapy—if it were available—to fix any genetic abnormalities in their children?

REFERENCES AND SUGGESTED READING

1. G.E. Wolstenhome and Maeve O'Connor, eds., *Ethics in Medical Progress* (Ciba Foundation) (Boston: Little, Brown and Company, 1966), p. 134. Hamberger's quotation is from J. Rostand, *Pensees d'un Biologiste* (Paris: 1939).
2. "Frances" is a pseudonym for a person interviewed by Lois Wingerson in **Mapping Our Genes** (New York: Plume, 1991).
3. "Huntington's Gene Finally Found," *Science* 260 (2 April 1993).
4. Jeremy Rifkin, *Algeny* (New York: Viking Press, 1983).
5. Robert Bazell, "Virus," *The New Republic* (9 November 1992).
6. For a good explanation of the history of sickle-cell anemia laws, see Phillip Reilly, *Genetics, Law and Social Policy* (Cambridge, MA: Harvard University Press, 1977), 62–86.
7. C.H. Sinnette, and J.A. Smith, eds., *Legislative and Socioeconomic Aspects of Sickle Cell Disease* (New York: Harlem Hospital Center, 1973).
8. Plato's *Republic.*
9. Christopher Marlowe, *Dr. Faustus* (New York: Signet Books, 1969).
10. *Time,* 4 January 1993.
11. Peter Medawar, *The New Genetics and the Future of Man,* ed. Michael Hamilton (Grand Rapids, MI: William Erdmans Publishing Co. 1972), 100. Quoted in Joseph Fletcher, *Ethics of Genetic Control* (New York: Anchor Books, 1974).
12. "A Speeding Ticket for NIH's Controversial Cancer Star," *Science,* 259 (5 March 1993).

CHAPTER 11

Justice and the Allocation of Scarce Resources

Instructional Goal

The major instructional goal for this chapter is to gain an understanding of our current national health care crisis, and to examine potential solutions under the principle of justice.

Instructional Objectives

At the end of this chapter the reader should understand and be able to:

1. Differentiate between Medicare and Medicaid as national programs.
2. Discuss how our current system of prospective payment and diagnostic related groups is an attempt to contain health care costs in the United States.
3. Identify three forces in our society that have tended to cause the dramatic inflation of health care costs in the United States.
4. Define and differentiate between micro allocation and macro allocation as they relate to health care.
5. Define and differentiate between formal and material justice.
6. State how the Fair Opportunity Rule relates to material justice.
7. Define and differentiate between the theoretical positions of utilitarianism, egalitarianism, and libertarianism as they relate to distributive justice.
8. Define and give examples of how medical and social utility are used in the micro allocation of scarce resources.
9. Discuss the process of "life boat ethics" and relate it to our dealings with Third World Nations.
10. Discuss the process of triage, and relate it to the micro allocation of beds in the intensive care units.

Glossary

Diagnostic Related Groups: Disease conditions have been gathered into related groups for determination of payment through the prospective payment system.

Distributive Justice: Refers to just distribution in society, structured by various moral, legal, and cultural rules and principles.

DNR Order: "Do Not Resuscitate" order; placed in charts of those patients who would not benefit from or do not desire cardiopulmonary resuscitation.

Egalitarian Allocation: A system of allocation that seeks to provide all things equally.

Fair Opportunity Rule: No person shall receive goods and services on the basis of an undeserved advantage nor be denied goods and services on the basis of an undeserved disadvantage.

Formal Justice: The ethical concern of formal justice is that the criteria are applied equally to all similar cases. Formal justice does not tell us whether the criteria are relevant or ethically valid, only that they are equally applied.

Libertarian Allocation: A system of allocation that is generally based on the free market exchange of goods and services.

Material Justice: The ethical concern of material justice is that the criteria used in allocation be relevant and ethically valid.

Medicaid: The national health program that provides health care for the poor.

Medical Utility: The allocation of scarce resources to those with the best prognosis.

Medicare: The national health program that provides health care for the elderly.

Prospective Payment: Medicare and Medicaid payments to hospitals are predetermined by diagnosis. The government is willing to pay only this predetermined fixed amount regardless of other circumstances.

Rights: An obligation based on the principle of justice, e.g., you have a right to your personal property.

Social Utility: The allocation of scarce resources to those who are most useful or valued by the society.

Triage: A system that divides the patient cases into categories so that care can be allocated effectively.

Utilitarian Allocation: A system of allocation that attempts to maximize public utility.

HEALTH CARE IN THE UNITED STATES

> *O health! health! The blessing of the*
> *rich! The riches of the poor! Who can buy*
> *thee at too dear a rate, since there is*
> *no enjoying this world without thee?*

Ben Johnson, Volpone, Act ii

We have come to ever more desire what we
cannot any longer have in unlimited
measure—a healthier, extended life—
and cannot even afford to pursue much
longer without harm to our personal lives
and other social institutions.[1]

Daniel Callahan, Director/Cofounder of the Hastings Center

Perhaps the most common characteristic of the "good life" as it is defined by any of the world's people, is good health. Health is valued above almost all other factors, such as wealth, education, or social status. A 1987 Harris Poll indicated that more than 90 percent agreed with the statement that "everyone should have the right to get the best possible health care—as good as the treatment a millionaire gets." Health care spending per family each year is approximately $6,535, of which two-thirds ($4,296) is paid out by the families, and one-third ($2,239) is paid by businesses. The cost of health care in 1992 jumped by 11 percent to $817 billion—or 14 percent of the gross national product (GNP). It is estimated that, if current spending trends continue, by the year 2020 health care spending could consume as much as 36 percent of the GNP, or one dollar out of every three. Our current spending of about one billion dollars per day for health care makes ours the costliest health care system per capita in the world today.[2]

In many areas of the economy, American industry and applied science have been eclipsed by our competitors, but medical science and technology is nowhere better developed than in our superb urban tertiary centers. Our National Institute of Health is one of the world's premier biomedical research organizations, with an annual budget of over $7 billion. We have more physicians per capita than most other industrialized nations, and health issues such as weight, smoking, exercise, drinking, and personal hygiene, are daily fare for our print and electronic news media. And although this generation of Americans is the healthiest ever, the actual improvement in health has not been matched by a subjective sense of better health. We live longer and better, yet as a nation we report more frequent and longer episodes of serious acute illness than citizens in the past. It appears that we have lowered the threshold for mild disorders and now are quicker to see in minor discomforts the signs of serious disease. We have become, in some sense, a nation of the worried well.

HEALTH CARE CRISIS

Yet, in the United States, there is a feeling of crisis in regard to health care. Even given our great financial outlays, we rank seventeenth in the world in infant mortality, and fifteen other nations have a life expectancy equal to or greater than ours. Nearly 38 million or about 15 percent of our citizens have neither private insurance nor government health care benefits.[3] In 1987, one out of five Americans had no insurance at some point during the year, as they were either unemployed or under employed and in a situation where benefits were not supplied by their employers. Disparities between the rich and poor, black and white have become more pronounced as infant mortality among African Americans is twice that of whites and early death from cancer and heart disease and other illnesses is more common in the poor than in the population as a whole. African Americans, who make up a disproportionate portion of the poor, have a life expectancy of 69.4 years compared to 75.4 years for whites.[4]

Although 90 percent of our citizens believe that everyone should have the best possible health care—equivalent to that available to a millionaire—a poll by the Public Agenda Foundation found that only one person in ten would accept a $125.00 tax increase to support a national insurance program for catastrophic illness. The concern over health care has grown until it is now a major issue in the national elections and in collective bargaining negotiations as companies seek to control the runaway costs of this fringe benefit.

In the affluent 1960s, voters authorized and supported increased expenditures for health care. Two titles were added to the Social Security Act of 1965, which increased reimbursement for health benefits from the federal government. Title XVIII established the **Medicare** program for the elderly. The second, Title XIX, the **Medicaid** program, expanded financial assistance which enabled states to pay medical services for the poor. Both of these titles allowed for hospitals to be reimbursed for the accrued costs of the care. Hospitals and health care providers were compensated for whatever care they provided, with no built-in incentives for cost containment. By the early 1980s, it became evident that the lack of controls in regard to health care costs were bringing the Medicare program to the brink of bankruptcy, and a new system was needed to stave off disaster. In 1983, a system of **prospective payment** was put into place. This system was not based on the traditional fee for service, rather, it paid a fixed fee per **diagnostic related group.** Because payment for a given illness was predetermined and fixed, health care facilities had a powerful incentive to contain costs. The most common forms of cost containment efforts were centered around reducing services, decreasing staff, and shortening the length of patient stay. The patients were in effect being sent home "sicker and quicker."

Even with massive governmental intervention, the spiral in health care costs continued. Many of these increases were fueled by our dependence on and successful use of lifesaving technology. Another factor is the change in the service population, as patients requiring hospital care are generally sicker and older (half over the age of 75) than in the past. The AIDS population is doubling every 9 to 12 months, and by 1992, AIDS care cost about $10 million per year.[5] Recent research reported in the Journal of the American Medical Association predicts that the care of babies born to cocaine-using mothers will create extra hospital costs of $504 million per year.

The Medicaid program, which pays for acute and long-term care for 27 million of our nation's poor, is the fastest-growing portion of state budgets. In 1980, it consumed about 9 percent of the state budgets and this had risen to 14% by 1991. In response to these spiraling costs, many states have tightened eligibility standards and cut benefits.[6]

The Medicare program in 1990 consumed about 61 cents of each federal health care dollar. It is projected that, if current trends continue, the expenditures threaten the solvency of the Medicare Hospital Insurance Trust Fund. The Advisory Council on Social Security has warned that the trust fund could go bankrupt by the year 2020.

Applied technology has decreased the mortality of infants and elongated the life expectancy of the general population. These changes can be clearly seen in the life expectancy of babies with birthweights below 2 lb. 3 oz. Prior to 1975, only 6 percent managed to live. By the mid 1980s, this figure had climbed to 48 percent. This technological success, however was bought at a staggering financial and physical price. One recent study done in regard to these tiniest of premature infants found that the average cost of care was $160,000, and that despite the extraordinary measures used, half of the surviving infants faced a lifetime of disabilities.[7]

Citizens have grown to expect miracles from medicine and, as a result, will often demand transfer from smaller hospital units to the more technologically advanced tertiary care centers. Whereas, in most other industries, the application of technology has been coupled with a decrease in the work force as labor-saving devices have been implemented, in health, technology has lead to further increases in the work force as each new technological application has seemingly justified a new set of health care specialists. Respiratory care, sonography, and perfusionism are relatively new specialties that owe their presence on the medical team to the technological advances of the last half century.

Middle-class citizens in the 1990s find themselves in a situation where personal income is dropping in a relative sense for most families, and both husband and wife must now work outside the home to maintain a stable quality of life. These citizens live in fear of catastrophic illness, or a change in work status that would reduce their insurance and place them outside the health care lifeboat. It is in this atmosphere of uncertainty that questions regarding health care distribution are being debated. There is a general feeling that we are entering a watershed period of change, but no consensus has yet been achieved. Our current dilemma is clearly stated by a recent author who wrote,

> We are at present committed to providing the best of care, equally to all, while maintaining provider and receiver choice, though at the same time engaging in cost containment. It should be clear that one cannot pursue all of these four goals at the same time. We confront a conflict of values and goals.[8]

MICRO AND MACRO ALLOCATION OF HEALTH CARE

The United States faces questions involving health care distribution at both the **macro allocation** and **micro allocation** level. Macro allocation is usually the province of congress, state legislatures, insurance companies, private foundations, and health organizations as the society attempts to determine how much should be expended and what kinds of goods and services will be made available. Macro allocation problems are demonstrated in such questions as: What kinds of health care will be available? Who will get it and on what basis? How will the costs be distributed? Who will deliver the services? Who controls these issues? Micro allocation is the more personal determination of who will receive scarce resources, such as intensive-care beds, advanced technology, or organ transplants.

FORMAL AND MATERIAL JUSTICE

The fair and equitable division of scarce goods and services is usually considered an issue of **distributive justice.** The requirements of **formal justice,** as attributed to Aristotle, are that in distribution, "equals must be treated equally, and unequals must be treated unequally." Formal justice does not attempt to provide any criteria for the determination of equality, nor does it state in what respect equals are to be treated, except that they must be treated equally. Under formal justice, any criteria could be used; age, sex, marital status, land ownership, provided the criteria was applied equally in all similar cases. Principles that specify relevant characteristics or determine morally relevant criteria in regard to treatment are said to be material principles and form the basis of **material justice.**

Society has used a wide variety of criteria for the distribution of resources. Figure 11–1 lists the common methods, but certainly does not exhaust the list of possible criteria.[9]

The ethically least acceptable rationing schemes would be those that placed individuals or groups disadvantaged by poverty or incapacitated by illness in the lowest priority. "Discrimination between classes of people is morally justified only if properties of the groups are the moral responsibility of the group members or if they are the sort of properties that can be overcome.[10]" This attempt to treat all equally is formulated in the **Fair Opportunity rule,** which holds that no persons should be granted social benefits on the basis of undeserved advantage, and that no persons should be denied social benefits on the basis of undeserved disadvantages. Under the fair opportunity rule, sex, race, IQ, national origin, sexual preference, and social status would be ruled out as relevant criteria for material justice in the moral distribution of health care.

THEORIES OF JUSTICE

In the debate over the allocation of health care resources, several theoretical positions have been advanced. Some have called for a total abandonment of governmental intervention, with goods and services being distributed by the invisible hands of a free market. They argue that the increases in health care costs, even in the face of massive governmental efforts to contain expenditures, threaten to break the back of

---

To each person an equal share
To each person according to need
To each person according to merit
To each person according to contribution
To each person according to effort
To each person according to social worth

FIGURE 11–1 Common Methods for the Distribution of Goods and Resources

the United States economy. These free-market disciples feel that the interventions themselves are the root of the problem and that if the government would cease all efforts to manipulate the market the price of health care would find its natural level. They point to research done by groups such as the Rand Corporation that seems to indicate that persons who have access to free health care use significantly more care than those who paid at least 25 percent of the costs.[11]

On the other extreme are there those who argue that an affluent society such as ours must find a way to pay health care costs. This group holds that members of the society are bound in a social contract, and that the presence of human need in the form of illness creates a moral obligation on the whole of the society. The society then has a collective obligation to provide these goods and services to the extent of its available resources.

Both of these positions, whether to place distribution in the hands of the free market, or to collectively provide services on the basis of social responsibility, will borrow aspects from one or more of three theoretical positions: **egalitarianism, utilitarianism,** or **libertarianism.**

Egalitarian Theories

These theories emphasize equal access to goods and services. In some of its more radical forms, egalitarianism holds that any deviations from absolute equality in distribution are unjust. However, this is a rather ideal formulation and does not correlate well with the reality of most situations governing the distribution of health care. A more useful formulation of egalitarianism can be found in the contract theory of John Rawls,[12] who holds that a social arrangement is an agreed-upon contract to advance the good of all who are in the society. In this communal effort, all would work toward the equal distribution of goods and services, unless an unequal distribution would work to everyone's advantage. Beauchamp and Childress have argued that this collective social protection and the **fair opportunity rule** form the basis of a right to health care.[13]

Utilitarian Theories

These theories emphasize a mixture of criteria so that public utility is maximized. Public utility is defined in the phrase "the greatest good for the greatest number." Utilitarians generally accept political planning and intervention as methods of redistributing goods and wealth to bring about public utility. The public health policies of many western nations have been formulated according to utilitarian theory. Many authorities, such as former Governor of Colorado Richard Lamm, see health care as just one of many human needs that must be served by public utility and feel that "We are treating our illnesses at the expense of our livelihoods. We spend more than a billion dollars a day for health care while our bridges fall down, our teachers are underpaid, and our industrial plants rust."[14] If our resources are limited and choices need to be made, does it make sense that in many of our cities the most technologically advanced area is the hospital and the least advanced our public schools?

Authorities such as Lamm and Daniel Callahan, Director of the Hastings Center, feel that even in times of moderate shortages of goods and services among societies, health care must be rationed and provided only to those who will benefit most and denied to those who will benefit less, such as the elderly. An example of this approach can be seen in Great Britain, where there exists a social, political, and medical consensus that allows practitioners to deny frail or severely demented elderly patients hospitalization or intensive care, even for such treatable conditions as pneumonia. It is considered reasonable, however, in Great Britain to provide extensive home care and geriatric day care. Not all theorists agree that health can be considered as other goods and many agree with Paul Ramsey that in a pluralistic society such as ours, placing health in conflict with better roads, schools, and bridges would be "almost, if not altogether, incorrigible to moral reasoning."[15]

One example of how a utilitarian rationing system might work has been proposed by Daniel Callahan and is known as the **natural life span argument**[16]. He feels that such a rationing scheme is necessary to stave off the ever-widening gap between resources and our expanding health needs caused by the flaws in our current system, as well as the increased needs generated by an aging population. Callahan argues that a natural life span is one that ends with a natural death and that this occurs at the end of the life cycle. Figure 11–2 lists the criteria used to establish the end of a natural life cycle. Using this theory, one can imagine allocating resources for oneself over the whole of one's life. One could devote, say, 10 percent to one's prenatal care, 10 percent to birth and early childhood, 10 percent to adolescence, 10 percent to years 20 through 40, and so on. We can see that such an allocation could be argued as rational and moral. Possibly it can be determined, for example, that money spent on the early years of one's life can make one's medical costs much less in later life. But one might also wish to concentrate one's expenditures in the twilight years to better "rage against the dying of the light," in the words of Dylan Thomas. If one could imagine allocating health care funds in this way for oneself, then it is not a large step to say that government would be justified in allocating health funds in a similar fashion. Indeed, it is quite likely that government could do a good job of allocating these funds, given all the statistical analysis that is available for health care expenditures over time.

We presently concentrate the largest portion of our health care dollar in the last years of people's lives. In 1990, the United States spent an estimated $661 billion on health care. It is estimated that within the population served by Medicare, 27.9 percent of the dollars spent were consumed by the 5.9 percent of the enrollees who died in that year.[17] We might decide that this is the best policy for humane reasons, but we might also decide that this is an inefficient use of limited health care funds.

Natural life then, would culminate in natural death (most often between 78 and 82 yrs), natural death should be accepted, and no life-extending technologies should be instituted. Callahan offers the following principles for practice: (1) After a person has lived out a normal life span, medical care should no longer be oriented to resisting death. (2) Medical care following a natural life span would be limited to relief of suffering. (3) The existence of technologies capable of extending life beyond a normal life span creates no technological imperative for its use.

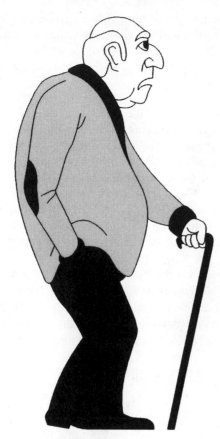

1. One's life work is completed.
2. One's moral obligations to those for whom one has responsibility have been discharged.
3. One's death does not seem to others an offense to sense or sensibility or tempt others to despair and rage at human existence.
4. When the process of dying is not marked by unbearable and degrading pain.

FIGURE 11–2 The End of a Natural Life Cycle

Those who have argued against the natural life span argument have done so using several lines of reasoning. First, there are questions in regard to the artificiality of setting a certain age range as constituting the natural life span, and second, Callahan has been somewhat vague in regard to what constitutes life-extending technologies. Under the model, a patient who was receiving a life-extending drug such as insulin prior to entry into the selected age group could continue until death. However, someone who began to need the drug in order to extend life—after completion of a natural life span—would have it denied.[18]

For all its faults, the life span model may be ethically persuasive if it operates as a closed system, where all savings gained from the limitation of technology at the end of your life would be used to enhance health during the other phases of natural life. The closed-system approach would assist in diminishing our current problems of intergenerational inequity, where one age group seems to benefit at the expense of others. As an example, our current federal expenditure for children is only one-sixth the outlay for the elderly, even though a greater number of children live in poverty.

With a closed system, moneys saved from providing life-extending technologies could be used to invest in childhood health and provide better maintenance for the elderly.

Libertarian Theories

Libertarians emphasize personal rights to social and economic liberty. They are not as concerned with, nor do they outline the requirements of, how the material goods and services are to be distributed, only that the choice of allocation system be freely chosen. In the United States, outside of our charity, social welfare, and military medical services, we have chosen for the most part to allocate health care goods and services using the free-market approach. Figure 11–3 provides one humorous vision of a libertarian future under "managed competition." The free-market approach has recently been criticized, as it has created not a unified system of health care delivery within our nation but a whole series of micro systems, some of which work well and others that appear broken.

Our free-market system that operates on the material principle of ability to pay usually invokes some form of libertarianism as its justification. Given our national penchant for personal liberty and individuality, it is quite likely that some aspects of the free market will coexist within any national health care plan we evolve.

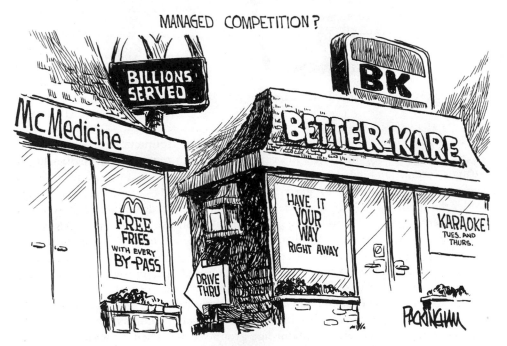

FIGURE 11–3

TWO-TIER SYSTEM AND THE DECENT MINIMUM

One interesting position in regard to the allocation of health care goods and services is that of the two-tier system. Under this approach, everyone would be guaranteed coverage for basic care and catastrophic health needs. This coverage of a decent minimum of care would be distributed on the basis of need, with everyone being assured equal access to basic and catastrophic services. The second tier, based on the ability to pay, would provide expanded and perhaps better care at private expense. This blending of utilitarian and libertarian values may have real appeal in the United States as we attempt to increase the services for those citizens who do not compete well in the marketplace.

THE OREGON RATIONING SYSTEM

One plan that is approaching the concept of a two-tier system is the Oregon rationing system, which was put into place to extend the benefits of health care to a wider population. In 1983, in response to a desire to expand the number of Oregonians who received an acceptable level of medical care, the state began to hold public meetings in regard to health policy. These meetings culminated in formation of a group known as the Citizens Health Care Parliament, which produced two reports: "Society Must Decide," and "Quality of Life in Allocating Health Care Resources." The Oregon Health Services Commission, using complicated cost-benefit analysis, set out to assess the relative value attached to each medical service by the citizens of the state. Each service was ranked on three factors: the public's perception of value, the effectiveness or outcome, and cost. The prioritization was to have the effect of denying some medically important treatments to Medicaid recipients. By decreasing the expenditures, the cost savings could be used to increase the number of people who could be served. The services considered most valuable on the basis of public perception, effectiveness and cost, were prenatal care, and those least valued were those involving infertility and cosmetic surgery. The goal was to expand the number of citizens eligible for care, by not providing every conceivable service of modern medicine. The 1988 legislature acted on these initiatives, making Oregon the first jurisdiction to explicitly decide on a rationing system for health care in the United States.[19] In the heat of the 1992 election, the administration placed a hold on the Oregon plan claiming that the rationing system was potentially discriminatory. The Clinton administration has been working on a national system of health care using a "managed competition" model. With a unified national system in place it is unclear where state models such as the Oregon system will fit.

There are those who argue that nothing should be rationed and everyone should be provided with everything. Why can't we have it all? (Let's have our cake and to eat it, too.) It has been projected that by the year 2020, if current trends continue, we will be spending 36 cents out of every dollar in the United States on health care.

Because this appears to be unworkable, our situation in health is somewhat akin to the ethics of the lifeboat, in that there are far too many citizens in need of services and too few services available.

LIFEBOAT ETHICS

In 1842, the American ship the *William Brown* struck an iceberg near Newfoundland and began to sink. The crew and half the passengers managed to leave the vessel in two overcrowded life boats. After 24 hours, one of these vessels began to founder in the high seas. The crew became concerned that all the lives would be lost unless they decreased the numbers in the boat. The decision was to give priority to married men and all women. Under this system, fourteen single men were thrown overboard, and two young women, sisters of men in the water, chose to join them. Several hours later, the survivors in the lifeboat were rescued by passing vessels.

Upon their return to Philadelphia, all of the crew—with the exception of Seaman Holmes—disappeared. Holmes was brought before the court to face trial for murder of the individuals thrown overboard. The defense argued that the actions were needed to save lives and that there were no volunteers to enter the water. The defense justified the decisions using the utilitarian value of keeping families intact and the duty-oriented value of protecting helpless females. The court, using a different duty-oriented approach based on the sacred nature of each life, stated that a lottery would have been the only ethical method, and Seaman Holmes was convicted.[20] This view that a random selection among equals is the best approach has been forcefully restated in the works of the ethicist, Paul Ramsey:

> the equal right of every human being to live, and not relative personal or social worth, should be the ruling principle. When not all can be saved and all need not die, this ruling principle can be applied best by random choice among equals.[21]

Lifeboat ethics, which take their title from this episode, have often been used to describe the situation of the industrialized western nations and their relationship to much of the third world. With seemingly more and more of the world's population living in conditions of famine and pestilence, we can see an analogy to a lifeboat afloat on a human sea of tragedy. Who shall be saved from drowning, and what will be the criteria for our selection?

TRIAGE

Similar in some aspects to lifeboat ethics is the process of **triage.** This process of allocating scarce resources has been commonly practiced and justified in the crises of war or disaster. When used in time of war, the practice is usually to divide the wounded into three groups. The first group is the walking wounded, who have received superficial wounds that require minimal care. These soldiers are often ignored during the first few minutes, or patched up immediately if they can be sent back to the battlefield. The second group are the fatally wounded, who are given available narcotics to ease their pain but are not treated for their injuries. The third group are the seriously wounded. These are treated immediately, as their care will bring about the highest percentage of survivors.

Similar principles to triage are used in the allocation of ICU beds when there is overcrowding. One criterion often used and very similar to those employed on the battlefield is that of best prognosis or **medical utility.** Which patient is most likely to survive? It is from this criterion that questions emerge as to whether patients with a **DNR order** truly belong in intensive care, if in fact we do not intend to treat them intensively.[22] A second common principle is **social utility,**—which patient has the greatest social worth. When the President of the United States is in any major United States city, critical trauma specialty areas are held in reserve in case of an emergency. His value to us as a society gives him a first call on these resources, based on the principle of social worth. However, both social utility and medical utility have inherent problems. Medical utility, or best prognosis, is often difficult to assess; and social utility, or social value decisions, seems to invite problems of racism, ageism, sexism, and bias against the retarded and mentally ill. Perhaps the most neutral system is that of "first come, first served," or random selection that treats all patients as essentially equal.

One interesting (although disturbing) experience with micro allocation through the criterion of social worth was the use of anonymous committees to determine who could be placed on kidney dialysis in the early 1960s, when the need for the therapy far outstripped the number of units available. In Seattle, these committees used factors such as age, sex, marital status, number of dependents, net worth, income, educational background, future potential, and emotional stability to make their decisions. It was interesting to note that if the individuals were later divorced, became alcoholics, or had financial downturns, they were not taken off the therapy, although they then did not match the criteria. Due to the lack of neutrality of the criteria, the committees' choices favored males, Caucasians, and the middle class or above. One critique quoted by Ramsey called the selection "a disturbing picture of the bourgeoisie sparing the bourgeoisie," and held that the "Pacific Northwest is no place for a Henry David Thoreau with bad kidneys."[23]

Although not as blatant as the Seattle experience, the difference between the moneys available for cardiac and pulmonary rehabilitation seems to be the result of social-worth criteria. The patient who suffers a cardiac arrest is usually younger than the pulmonary patient. Once cardiac patients have completed rehabilitation, they often return to their positions and again produce work and pay taxes. Pulmonary patients, however, are usually beyond their working years, and once rehabilitation is complete, patients may lead a better quality of life, but usually not one productive in work output or active in the payment of taxes. Both forms of rehabilitation seem needful and beneficial to the patients, however cardiac rehabilitation is more available, better funded, and more likely to receive third-party payer support.

SUMMARY

In the United States, although we have a very high standard of health care, inflationary rises in costs due to increased demands for services and the use of expensive life-extending technology threaten to overwhelm the system. In 1993, we were spending about 14 cents out of every dollar of the gross national product on health care, and the trend indicates increases in the foreseeable future. These costs have escalated, even in the face of massive governmental intervention by way of prospective payment. The end result of our seeming inability to contain costs has been to place an ever-increasing number of our citizens outside our health care system, without money to purchase care, insurance, or health benefits to cover costs. A recent study highlights the problems our system is facing: Uninsured infants, while having more severe medical problems, received fewer medical services than those provided to babies who were privately insured or cared for under Medicaid. This decline in quality of health care afforded to uninsured Americans seems pervasive across the whole system. A feeling of crisis permeates the nation in regard to health care issues as we struggle to decide who is entitled to what and who is to pay.

National discussions in regard to the micro and macro allocation of health care resources have centered around the principle of justice. Proponents of egalitarian, libertarian, and utilitarian theories of justice have put forward a variety of rationing schemes. Figures 11–4, 11–5, and 11–6 outline the three approaches under consideration following the 1992 election year. The options available range over the full spectrum of political philosophy. There are those who argue for a pure capitalist approach, whereby costs are contained by the invisible hands of a free market. Others see the need for a utilitarian system, with government distributing care so as to provide the best for the most by restricting access of certain therapies to selected patient groups. Still others admire egalitarian proposals, by which everyone has equal access to all the care available consistent with resources.

Several mixed models for the macro allocation of health care resources have been put forward. They call for a two-tiered system that provides a decent minimum level of basic and catastrophic care available to all citizens, using the criterion of need, and a second tier of more complete care available to those who can afford to purchase it. The concept of a two-tiered system, providing a decent minimum of care, forms the basis of the system still under consideration in Oregon.

On the micro allocation level, groups have struggled with the allocation of such diverse resources as mechanical hearts, fresh organs, and intensive-care beds. Several systems have been put forward, looking at a variety of triage schemes, with criteria based on such concepts as social and medical utility, ability to pay, first come first served, and the lottery. Whatever system is finally selected, to be ethically sound it must not fall more heavily upon the socially disadvantaged or those incapacitated by illness. The weighing of one class of treatments or technologies against another must take place in a closed system. When beneficial care is denied to one group it must be because there is a better use of those resources elsewhere in the system. The criteria for making decisions of what constitutes "better use" should be in accordance with

This approach seeks to build upon our existing system by encouraging everyone to buy health insurance with the assistance of tax credits, tax deductions, and redeemable vouchers. Some citizens would receive health insurance through purchasing it, others through their employers, and low-income individuals would receive tax credit/vouchers that would make health insurance affordable and available.

FIGURE 11–4 Private-market Approach

This approach calls for a national health insurance provided by the government. Everyone would receive access to a guaranteed basic hosptal and physician coverage. Employers would no longer be required to provide coverage for employees but would contribute financially to the universal health plan. Private health insurance companies would play no part in the plan, but might provide additional coverage through supplemental insurance.

FIGURE 11–5 Government-based Approach

Sometimes called the "play or pay" approach, this plan calls for employers to either "play" by providing health insurance for employees, or "pay" a tax that provides coverage through a public plan. Either way, everyone receives health insurance, either from an employer or the government. Medicare would still be in place for older citizens and those handicapped.

FIGURE 11–6 Employer-based Approach

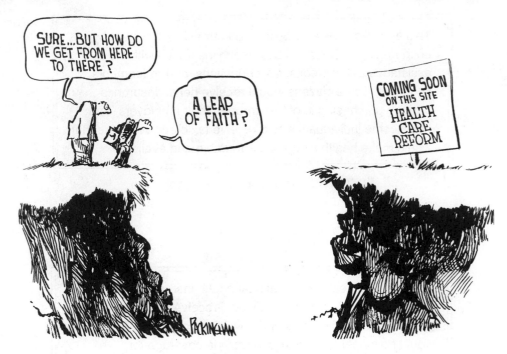

FIGURE 11—7

the principle of material justice, and the fair opportunity rule. These are difficult decisions and unfortunately Figure 11—7 accurately reflects our current state as we prepare to enter the next century.

CLARIFICATION EXERCISES

A. Our society has chosen several methods of resource allocation, such as: need, ability to pay, merit, potential worth, past contribution, and equal share. All of these could form the basis of distribution according to formal justice (as long as equals are treated equally, and unequals unequally). Which do you think is best suited for the requirements of material justice? Defend your answer.

   If you chose "need" as the basis for resource allocation, consider the following rejection of need as a criterion for just distribution drawn from the works of Ayn Rand[24].

   A morality that holds need as a claim, holds emptiness—nonexistence—as its standard of value; it rewards an absence, a defect: weakness, inability, incompetence, suffering, disease, disaster, the lack, the fault, the flaw, the zero. Who provides the account to pay these claims? Those who are cursed for being non-zero, each to the extent of his distance from that ideal. Since all values are the product of virtues, the degree of your virtue is used as the measure of your penalty; the degree of your fault is used as the measure of your gain.

The emphasis of Ayn Rand's statement is similar to the reasoning used against providing welfare payments for able-bodied persons, as they seem to be getting "Something for Nothing," while those who work are penalized for their efforts. What gives anyone the *right* to the services of health care providers, given that we do not claim any rights to the services of the butcher, banker, or baker?

Some 40 to 50 percent of Americans—the aged, children in poverty, the dependent poor, and those with chronic disabilities—require larger amounts of health care than they have the financial resources to purchase. Does their need provide a reasonable justification for their demand for service? Defend your answer.

B. With prospective payment, the charges that can be made for a particular condition are predetermined and fixed; hospitals make or lose money depending upon whether they are able to treat the patient within the confines of the predetermined payment. This has resulted in pressure on health care providers to reduce staff, reduce length of hospital stay, and reduce services provided. Can a health care provider serve both the society's need for cost containment and yet be the advocate for the patient as required by the basic principles of role duty and beneficence?

C. On September 21, 1971, an infant was born with severe combined immunodeficiency disease (SCID). The family and physicians involved, knowing that the baby had an even chance of having the fatal illness, had the child delivered by cesarean section and then sealed in a plastic chamber. Frequent newspaper reports on "David the bubble boy" continued through the years, as he was moved to larger and larger chambers. The absolute devotion of his family, coupled with approximately $200,000 per year in research grants from the National Institute of Health, and extraordinary and imaginative technology, allowed David to remained free from contact with organisms and to celebrate his twelfth birthday. After attempted treatment of bone marrow previously treated using monoclonal antibodies, David died on February 22, 1984.[25]

If David were born next week instead of in 1971, do you think that we should begin the ever-more-demanding bubble process? Whatever your answer, defend it using some rational ethical criteria.

D. The National Commission to Prevent Infant Mortality points out that for every $1 invested in prenatal care, $3–$10 is saved on post natal care. The nation spends about $2 billion a year on hospital care to keep low birth weight babies alive, and many of those who survive are left with a lifetime of medical disability. For a quarter of the cost spent on low birth weight babies, prenatal care could be provided to all pregnant women who now go without care.

Assuming that you could use the money saved by not providing for low birth weight babies on prenatal care for all women, as well as better "well baby" care for all infants, would you make the choice? Whatever your answer, defend it based on some criteria of justice.

E. In our society, African Americans do not donate organs at the same rate as do white Americans, and they have a higher rate of rejection of implanted organs. The difference in donation rate appears to be based on sociological factors such as poverty and religious beliefs. The reason for the higher rejection rate is unknown. Given the current scarcity of organs available for implantation, do you feel that black Americans should be denied equal access to available organs? Whatever your answer, defend your position according to some relevant criteria of material justice.

F. There are all types of patients who need liver transplants, ranging from those whose liver fails due to genetic problems or accidents to those who have destroyed their livers through the use of alcohol. Should a person who is currently an alcoholic have the same access to available livers as those who, through no fault of their own, need a liver transplant? Whatever your answer, defend your position according to some relevant criteria of material justice.

If your answer above was "no, the alcoholic should not get another liver," how would you feel about lungs for smokers, any organ for a drinker involved in an auto accident, hearts for fat people, etc.?

G. In the Oregon rationing system, the commission attempted to rank-order over 700 differing health care services on the basis of perception of value, effectiveness, and cost. Rank-order the following 20 services using these criteria. First, rank-order the list individually, then rank-order them as a group. In that some of the services may be of equal value to you, give them the same ranking (e.g., it will be possible to have more than one service in first or second place).

Once we have rank-ordered the list, we can often get a better discrimination between items by giving our choices a weight factor. This is done by first adding all of the individual rankings and then dividing this number by the total number of items, which in this case is 20. Each individual ranking is then divided by the factor to discriminate between items.

	Rank Order	Weight Value
1. Prenatal care		
2. Neonatal intensive care		
3. Mammography		
4. Cardiac rehabilitation		
5. Nursing home maintenance		
6. Genetic screening		
7. Pulmonary rehabilitation		
8. Well baby care		
9. Drug rehabilitation		
10. Liposuction		
11. Cosmetic surgery		
12. Organ transplants		
13. Burn centers		
14. Fertility clinics		
15. Primary care services		
16. Dietetics		
17. Sports medicine		
18. AIDS treatment centers		
19. Chemotherapy		
20. Dental and orthodontics		

H. Look at your top five weighted items and your bottom five weighted items. What, if anything, does it say about your perception of value? Would you say you were more favorable to any age group? Would you say that you had a bias toward social utility? How did drug rehabilitation and AIDS patients fare?

I. You have a four-bed intensive care unit and seven patients who need a bed. The following is a short description of the seven patients. You cannot select on the basis of "first come, first served," as they showed up at your door at exactly the same time.

1. Mr. Jones, a 75-year-old pulmonary patient with chronic emphysema. He is retired, and has a DNR (do not resuscitate) order.

2. Ms. Smith, a 27-year-old hemophiliac patient with AIDS contracted from a transfusion of contaminated blood.

3. Mr. Rogers, a 65-year-old retired general with congestive heart failure.

4. Mrs. Rankin, a 52-year-old housewife, and alcoholic, with acute liver disease.

5. Ms. Reubin, a 23-year-old college student, in a persistent coma following an alcohol/drug overdose at a party.

6. Carlton Child, a 12-year-old with head trauma, and in a persistent vegetative state, following a beating by his step-father.

7. Joey Scoy, a severely retarded Down's syndrome teenager, with a mental age of five years. He is suffering from aspiration pneumonia.

Select your four patients, and state what criteria you used to exclude the three.

J. Do patients with DNR orders belong in intensive care if there is a bed shortage? How would you make the decision as to who stays and who goes? Would you use medical utility, social utility, or an egalitarian "first come, first served"?

In 1990 about $30 billion in Medicare funds was spent on the 5 percent of Medicare patients who were in the last six months of life. This seemingly wasteful process is justified by the number of patients who are expected to die but who surprise physicians and live. Recently, there has been reported a computerized predictive system, known as APACHE III, that measures 28 physiologic variables used to determine objectively the probability of survival during the hospital stay.

If the APACHE system were able to predict with a 98 percent certainty those patients who would not survive, no matter how much intensive care they received, we might be able to save over $20 billion in public funding each year by ceasing to care for them intensively and to provide only palliative care. This would mean, however, that 2 percent of the patients who might have survived had we continued intensive care would not, although they would probably not have been long-lived regardless of our efforts.

How should society respond to these new computer predictive tools?

K. Some authorities, such as Daniel Callahan, argue that as long as we continue to focus on the individuals' needs and desires for health care resources we are doomed to failure as there is seemingly no end to what we individuals may require in postponing the inevitability of our mortality. If we as a society provided health care on the basis of what was needed for a healthy society, we might gain control over the expenditures for health.

In this section, outline what you think might be a requirement for a healthy society. e.g. "A healthy society needs enough workers to work well and hard to take care of their own needs and the needs of our society." In your answer, be sure that you provide for the national defense, democratic institutions, and an educated citizenry.

Given your descriptions of society's needs, would we need to provide heart transplants to those over 55, AZT for AIDS patients, or neonatal care for infants under 500 grams? Would the society benefit in any real sense by medical technology extending our life expectancy from the current 75 years to 95? Do you feel that moving from an individual needs-based system to a societal needs-based system makes sense? Write what you feel about such a proposal. Defend your ideas.

L. In this exercise, you will find three value statements in regard to health care delivery. Write three more statements that you can agree with.

1. The principle of justice should prevail in the distribution of health care.

2. Society has a moral obligation to care for the suffering.

3. Any system of health care delivery selected must not fall more heavily upon those least able to afford care.

M. Figures 11–4, 11–5, and 11–6 outline the basic health care reform packages being discussed in the nation today. Attempt to label them using the following political terms, egalitarian (socialist), utilitarian (liberal), or libertarian (conservative).

1. Private-market approach   _____

2. Government-based approach   _____

3. Employer-based approach   _____

State which of the three you support and why.

REFERENCES AND SUGGESTED READING

1. Daniel Callahan, *What Kind of Life* (New York: Simon and Schuster, 1990).
2. Ruth Purtilo, "Saying No to the Patients for Cost-Related Reasons," *Physical Therapy,* Physical Therapy Association 68, no. 8 (August 1988): 1243–1247.
3. Judith Rooks, "Let's Admit We Ration Health Care: Then Set Priorities," *American Journal of Nursing* (June 1990): 39–43.
4. Barbara Coombs, "Two Ethics Compete in Debate on Health Care Rationing," *Journal of the American Academy of Physicians Assistants* (Sept 1990): 436–438.
5. Kathleen Perrin, "Rationing Health Care" *Journal of Gerontological Nursing* 15, no. 9. (1989): 10–14.
6. Chris Wood, "Health Care Rationing: The Oregon Experiment," *Nursing Economics* 9, no. 4. (July/August 1991): 239–242.
7. "Should Every Baby Be Saved?" *Time* (June 1990).
8. H.T. Englehardt, "The Importance of Values in Shaping Professional Direction and Behavior," *Occupational Therapy Education: Target 2000,* American Occupational Therapy Association (1986): 40.
9. Gene Outka, *Social Justice and Equal Access to Health Care* in R. Veatch and R. Branson, eds., *Ethics and Health Policy* (New York: Ballinger Publishing Company, 1976), 79–91.
10. Tom Beauchamp and James Childress, *Principles of Biomedical Ethics* (New York: Oxford University Press, 1989), 271.
11. J. P. Newhouse, C. N. Corris, et al., "Some Interim Results from a Controlled Trial of Cost-Sharing in Health Insurance," *New England Journal of Medicine* 305 (1981): 1501–1507.
12. John Rawls, *A Theory of Justice* (Cambridge: Harvard University Press, 1971).
13. Beauchamp and Childress, *Principles of Biomedical Ethics,* p. 276.
14. Richard Lamm, "Rationing of Health Care: The Inevitable Meets the Unthinkable," *Nurse Practitioner* 11 no. 5 (1986): 581–583.
15. Paul Ramsey, *The Patient as a Person: Exploration in Medical Ethics* (New Haven: Yale University Press, 1970), 240.
16. Daniel Callahan, *Setting Limits: Medical Goals in an Aging Society* (New York: Simon and Schuster, 1987).
17. Peter Singer and Frederich Lowy, "Rationing, Patient Preferences, and the Cost of Care at the End of Life," *Archives of Internal Medicine* 152 (March 1992): 478–480.
18. Amitai Etzioni, "Spare the Old, Save the Young," *The Nation,* 11 June 1988.
19. Barbara Coombs, "Two Ethics Compete in Debate on Health Care Rationing," 1990.
20. *United States v. Holmes,* 26 Fed Cas 360 (CCED Pa 1842).
21. Barbara Edwards, "Does the DNR Patient Belong in the ICU?" *Critical Care Nursing Clinics of North America.* 2, no. 3 (Sept. 1990): 473–479.

22. Paul Ramsey, *The Patient as a Person: Exploration in Medical Ethics* (1970), 256.
23. Paul Ramsey, *The Patient as a Person: Exploration in Medical Ethics* (1970), 240.
24. Ayn Rand, *Atlas Shrugged* (New York: Signet Books, 1957), 958.
25. "Bubble Boy," editorial, *Journal of the American Medical Association* 253, no. 1 (4 Jan 1985).

CHAPTER 12

Professional Gatekeeping as a Function of Role Fidelity

Instructional Goal

Upon completion of this chapter the reader will understand how the requirements of professionalism lead to a whole series of gatekeeping tasks under the principle of role fidelity.

Instructional Objectives

At the end of this chapter the reader should understand and be able to:

1. List the rationale for a profession's creating a code of ethics.
2. State an ethically based rationale for forbidding sexual relations between patients and health care providers.
3. State an ethically based rationale for discouraging conflicts of interest in our practices.
4. Outline the importance of a scope of practice as it relates to practitioner activities.
5. Define disparagement, and state why it is a problem that is to be avoided in health care practice.
6. Outline the ethical obligation that we have toward impaired colleagues.

Glossary

Caveat emptor: The buyer beware.

Code Blue: One of many announcements used to signal an emergency team that assistance is needed for a cardiac arrest.

Disparagement: To belittle, or criticize the skill, knowledge, or qualifications of another professional.

Gatekeeping: A generic term used for a whole series of activities needed to protect the profession from those who would misuse the appropriate functions of that specialty. An example of the gatekeeping function might be the requirement that one professional report the misconduct of another.

Impaired Colleague: A colleague who can no longer function appropriately within the specialty. This may be due to illness or the use of substances such as alcohol or drugs.

Joint Venturing: In common usage, the situation in which a health professional has an investment interest in a health care facility.

Patient Advocate: To serve as the proponent of the patient's interests. This has become one of the important roles ascribed to the nursing profession.

Red-Tagged: A term used in the context of this chapter to indicate a "do not resuscitate" order.

Role Fidelity: To practice your professional role with full faithfulness.

Safe Harbor Rules: Rules that allow a questionable practice such as self-referral to continue due to the special circumstances of a particular case whereby the practice serves the patient's interests.

Scope of Practice: The tasks that are included within the practice of a specialty. Quite often the scope of practice is set forth in the legal regulations that allow the practice within a state.

Self-Referral: A term used to describe a health care provider's referral of patients to an outside facility in which he or she has a financial interest but no professional responsibility.

PROFESSIONAL GATEKEEPING AND PROFESSIONAL OBLIGATIONS

In his book Of Mice and Men, *John Steinbeck pointed out the decline in moral values when one of his characters commented, "There's nothing wrong anymore."*

There are two educations. One should teach us how to make a living and the other how to live.

John Truslow Adams

DISPARAGEMENT OF PROFESSIONAL COLLEAGUES

In practice, allied health and nursing personnel have long known that our physician colleagues were very loathe to criticize other physicians and practiced **gatekeeping** as part of their professional duties. This gatekeeping function, whereby one looks out for the interests of the profession or of others in a similar practice comes as a result of our professional obligations and training, which lead to a strong sense of collegiality with others in our practice. The following quote from the General Medical Council Handbook, *Professional Conduct and Discipline,* outlines the obligations of practitioners in regard to disparagement.

> It is improper for a doctor to disparage, whether directly or by implication, the professional skill, knowledge, qualifications, or service of any other doctor, irrespective of whether this may result in his own professional advantage, and such disparagement may raise a question of serious professional misconduct.[1]

Yet, as health care providers, we are often faced with the question raised by Cain: "Am I my brother's keeper?" As a member of a health profession the answer is often yes! Not only are we responsible for our actions in regard to the patient but we are also charged with the duty to assure that the rest of the health team is practicing appropriate care. The patients who are served have a certain vulnerability and dependence that is not usually found with other professional occupations. It is the essence of the therapeutic relationship and the trust that it inspires that makes individuals feel so betrayed and outraged when abuses occur.

Although some health care practitioners are independent entrepreneurs, the principle of **caveat emptor** cannot be allowed to govern the interactions between clients and health care providers. To protect vulnerable patients from exploitation, regulatory licensing mechanisms, legal remedies, and peer-review systems have come into being. The code of ethics that is part of each of our professions does more than set forth a series of ethical rules for the membership. It symbolizes that this group of professionals are differentiating themselves from the broader group of occupations and technical careers. One of the essential characteristics of a profession is that the members generate a code of ethics and are willing to become self regulating. It is true that sometimes codes of ethics serve rather crude ends, such as limiting competition, restricting advertising, and promoting a particular image, especially during the initial stages of professional development. The first American physician code, written in 1847, was directed as much toward separating orthodox practitioners from homeopaths, empirics, Thomsonians, and neuopaths, as it was toward regulating ethical conduct. Even in the modern codes of ethics, there is often a vagueness in both what one should do and what is to be avoided. Internally, there are often conflicts between the various prescriptive rules, and unresolved questions in regard to peer review and enforcement where conduct is found to be inappropriate. Still the main importance of a code of ethics is to affirm that the professional is an autonomous, responsible decision maker, not someone who just follows orders. There is an implied promise that the practitioner will not pursue his own interests at the expense of the client or patient. This implied promise then obligates the practitioner to the maintenance of professional gatekeeping in a great number of areas.

In the early 1980s, an allied health educator became disturbed by the number of ill-advised resuscitation efforts being called for in the local hospitals. In order to bring attention to the practice and to bring about needed reforms the therapist wrote the following article for his local society newsletter:[2]

A month or so ago, a young lady who had had two heart surgeries and a couple of (cardiac) arrests during the past two years, which resulted in hypoxic brain damage that had left her feeble minded and with a convulsive disorder, arrested again at home one evening because of a failed pacemaker. She was resuscitated and brought into the hospital, with no oxygen in the ambulance. There in the medical intensive care unit where everyone knew her from prior admissions, she arrested AGAIN about an hour later. Since she was not **red-tagged,** we were obliged to resuscitate her AGAIN, and put her on a ventilator. There she literally rotted away for three or four weeks (they had promptly fixed her pacemaker so that her heart wouldn't be able to stop again), until in spite of hell (which included dialysis for renal failure for over a week) she finally managed to "die."

Now, if one of the male staff had jumped into her bed and raped her, this would have been regarded as a criminal assault, and everyone would have been outraged, right? But what we did was far more damaging physically, far more protracted, and not one whit less immoral. Just the same, in the eyes of our curious social system, it was OK. Some system!

Another time recently I was privileged to attend a **code blue** on a patient who had arrested during cobalt therapy! That was only one of a whole series of resuscitations done routinely on terminal cancer patients at that hospital.

Why, when such patients have literally nothing going for them, must we be so hell-bent on interfering with this perfectly natural process which would relieve them of their hopeless suffering? Have our physicians taken complete leave of their senses? These are outrageous prostitutions of the art and science of resuscitation.

Resuscitation is the most literally lifesaving act the therapist performs. It is the noblest, loftiest, most heroic, and should be the most God-like thing one mortal can do for another. But everytime I am called to one of these grossly inappropriate codes, I am sick in my soul at this UN-godly, beastly business. The dictum that we are required to resuscitate ANYbody who arrests if he is untagged, no matter what's wrong with him or how long before he has been found the arrest may have occurred, really sticks in my craw. It is just reckless irresponsibility of the most irrational and immoral sort.

What's behind this tragedy? NEGLECT! Nobody talked with the patient or his family about whether he (they) wanted him resuscitated if he should arrest. Doubtless the rule always to do so in the absence of a **no code** order was put there because of the policy that nobody but a physician should make this decision. This can, of course, be construed as protecting nonphysicians from being accused of not resuscitating a patient who was in their judgment nonsalvageable.

But we all know of all too many instances where the doctor has specified NOTH-ING either way, and where the wishes of the patient or his family have NOT been explored. This situation is, of course, inescapable when there is no time; but usually the subject was just plain avoided because it was too unpleasant.

I think we should complain about this to our medical directors, and try to get them to use their influence on medical staffs to face this responsibility squarely, and then definitely to red tag or no code all patients who are either (a) not regarded as salvage-able, or (b) who have expressed their desire to be allowed to die in peace. Actually, hospitals could relieve doctors of some of this unpleasantry by making this question a part of the admissions interview with either the patient or the next of kin.

In terms of the earlier quote from the General Medical Council book on professional disparagement, the therapist—while perhaps in the right—was guilty of professional disparagement of his colleagues. The end result of the therapist's article as applied to inappropriate resuscitation was not a great change in clinical practice but rather harm to his own distinguished career. The point of the matter was not whether his account was untrue, or even whether he had an absolute right and perhaps a duty to bring it to the attention of the professional community. The problem lay in the manner of his presentation. Often, in questions of morals, we feel so intensely about what we consider to be right that we consider those who are in opposition to our point of view not merely wrong but evil. In the article, the therapist goes well beyond presenting a legitimate problem and likens the physicians' practice to criminal assault and rape. In assigning reasons for why the practice continued, his only rationales were that perhaps the physicians had taken leave of their senses, or were neglectful or recklessly irresponsible. It is not likely that such a manner of presentation would have gained him willing listeners among those he accused.

There are many problems in modern health care practice that need to be addressed, and the allied health practitioner and nurse have an important part to play in these discussions. The effectiveness of our input—that is, the willingness of others to listen and to cause positive change—will have a great deal to do with the collegiality of our presentation and the positive nature of our proposals.

CONFLICTS OF INTEREST

Recently, in the literature, health care provider joint-venturing and self-referral practices have been questioned. Most of these criticisms have been directed toward physicians who have joint-ventured into health care services such as physical therapy, diagnostic imaging centers, ambulatory surgical centers, and durable medical equipment companies. Simultaneously with these joint business interests has come an increase in outpatient costs, which appears to be linked to the practice of self-referral. Recent surveys in regard to this practice show that there is an apparent link between self-referral and increased costs, increased utilization, and reduced quality of care.[3] The degree of joint venturing is somewhat disturbing, as it is estimated by the Office of the Inspector General that 12 percent of the physicians who bill the Medicare program have ownership interests in health care firms to which they make referrals. Nationwide about 8 percent of physicians are involved in joint ventures. Data reported on the proportion of patient referrals by physician investors indicate that most of these facilities receive the majority of their referrals from physician owners.[4]

Obviously, in some or even a majority of these instances the patients are well served. In some cases, these joint ventures create a competitive atmosphere, and may even provide services to a community that might otherwise be unavailable. In these instances, the joint ventures serve a patient-centered health care ethic and perhaps **safe harbor rules** need to be put into place to allow these clinics to continue to function.

However, whether it serves a patient-centered ethic or no, self referral is suspect and causes a credibility gap that is hard to overcome. From the outside, joint venturing appears to be a practice "where one comes to do good and winds up doing well." In response to these criticisms, the American Medical Association recently adopted a new policy against physician self-referral. The policy holds that, in general, physicians should not refer patients to health care facilities where they have an investment interest but do not themselves provide direct medical service.[5]

It seems clear that to self-refer to an establishment where you do not provide service but have an economic interest is at least suspect and perhaps unethical. Yet there are other equally serious situations of conflict of interest that are more subtle. What of the pens, writing pads, free texts, medical equipment, and drug samples that at times seem a normal part of the delivery of health care? Does the fact that the gift is small make it more ethical to receive? An estimated 165 million dollars is spent each year by drug companies to influence physicians in regard to their purchases. Where does this process of receiving goods from drug firms or equipment companies cease to be good advertisement and begin to be unethical? If you were invited to a free seminar held on a cruise ship—where your travel, housing, food, and entertainment were picked up by a company—would this be unethical or continuing education? In one case, physicians were asked to participate in a drug study. The drug that was being studied offered no substantive therapeutic advantage over other drugs of its class and was somewhat more expensive. The doctors were reimbursed $125 for each patient they enrolled in the study, to cover their time and expenses.[6] Did that represent a bribe or gratuity or was it a legitimate reimbursement to otherwise busy professionals who had done the company a service and participated in important research? Do these practices affect patient care in regard to what companies the patients were referred to, or what pharmaceuticals were used? If the practices did change the behavior on the part of the health care practitioner, was the change brought about on the basis of new information gained, or favors granted? The very fact that such questions can be asked should cause professional concern.

Although much has been written in regard to the joint venturing practices of physicians and their relationships with drug companies, it is very difficult to determine exactly where the line should be drawn. Reflections on these same practices can be found in the dealings of nursing and allied health professionals. How many of the national, state, and local meetings that these practitioners attend are underwritten by commercial companies? To stem the practice of therapists referring their recently hospitalized patients to local durable medical equipment companies and receiving a finder's fee, the respiratory care national association (AARC) has been very vigorous in its condemnation of referrals whereby the practitioner had monetary gain.[7] Figure 12–1 outlines the AARC statement. Conflict of interest is not limited to the practice of physicians, and is equally suspect as a practice whoever the health care provider. A practitioner who changes his way of practice through any motive other than patient benefit has embarked on a slippery slope of compromised ethics. As a patient care provider, each professional will need to evaluate and

> The Code of Ethics of the AARC applies to all respiratory care practices regardless of the environment in which care may be delivered. In general, the following definition of conflict of interest is provided:
>
> Under no circumstances should any respiratory care practitioner engage in any activity which compromises the motive for the provision of any therapy procedures, the advice or counsel given patients and/or families, or in any manner profit from referral arrangements with home care providers.

FIGURE 12–1 AARC Statement Regarding Ethical Performance of Respiratory Home Care

prioritize to determine the point at which a service or provided gift ceases to be merely good advertisement, or continuing education, and begins to be a favor offered to compromise the client-centered nature of our health care practice.

SEXUAL MISCONDUCT IN HEALTH CARE PRACTICE

> Whatever houses I may visit, I will come for the benefit of the sick, remaining free of all intentional injustice, of all mischief and in particular of sexual relations with both female and male persons, be they free or slave.
>
> *Hippocratic Oath*

It is generally held among all health care providers that sexual relations between practitioners and patients are unethical. This is true because the relationship between practitioner and patient is always unequal. The nature of the practitioner/patient relationship places the practitioner in a position of advantage in the critical areas of knowledge, power, status, and personal vulnerability. Often, very intimate relationships are formed on the basis of our roles, and these can be powerful and intense for both patient and practitioner alike. Moreover, these normal, caring relationships developed between provider and patient frequently evoke strong and complicated feelings. These emotions of admiration, caring, and trust can be misunderstood, and patients are especially vulnerable when they are experiencing intense pressures or major traumatic life events.

Because of these inequalities of position, sexual relations under these situations cannot be considered, nor can they be understood as representing the true consent on the part of the patient. Inasmuch as practitioners have an obligation to treat the needs of the patient first, their own personal gratification cannot become a consideration. The therapeutic relationship rests on the patient's belief that the health care provider is dedicated to her welfare and that there are no other motives or considerations. Sexual relations, by their very nature, create emotional factors that interfere with the therapeutic relationship and the needed objective judgment. Whether due to a temporary failure to manage the therapeutic relationship, or due to crass exploitation of a professional situation, these relationships are neither ethically excusable nor condonable.

When the practitioner feels that a potential for misunderstanding is possible, or when he feels that there is the potential for mutual feelings of romantic interest, it is time to end the professional relationship. In that the patient's feelings formed during a time of illness often extend beyond the health care situation, the termination of care does not in itself provide an ethical basis for such a relationship to blossom into sexual contact. If the practitioner is exploiting the feelings of regard, respect, trust, and vulnerability gained as a result of the patient/provider relationship, the ethical propriety of such action is still suspect. In regard to the obvious question of how long is an acceptable period of interruption of the association, the answer is whatever time it takes, until the emotions derived from the relationship cannot be misused or manipulated.

Scope of Practice

All allied health and nursing personnel work within a **scope of practice.** This scope of recognized duties for our professions is usually set by the traditions of our specialty and/or by state legislation that enables our practice. Figure 12–2 lists the elements usually found in a scope of practice act. Practitioners who stray outside the scope of legitimate duties not only call upon themselves censorship from their peers and colleagues but also may face loss of legal credentials or litigation. The principle of **role fidelity** requires that we remain within our scope of legitimate practice. In most cases, the scope of practice is clear, and one does not cross the line without willful intention. For example, the nursing or allied health practitioner who is performing physicals and pretending to be a physician has not made an honest error. However, traditions and practices change, and sometimes the line is not as clear as one might suppose.[8] The following case outlines the problems that can occur as a result of being unclear as to specific duties, especially during a period in which there is a shift of traditional roles.

Practice acts will vary in emphasis but the majority will address the following elements:

    a. Scope of professional practice

    b. Requirements and qualifications for licensure

    c. Exemptions

    d. Grounds for administrative action

    e. Creation of an examination board and processes

    f. Penalties and sanctions for unauthorized practice

FIGURE 12–2 Basic Elements of a Practice Act

In the mid-70s, a nursing educator in Idaho had contact, through a student, with a female client who had chronic myelogenous leukemia. This form of leukemia can often be managed for years with little or no chemotherapy. The woman had done well for 12 years and had ascribed her good health to health foods and a strict nutritional regime. However, her condition had turned for the worse several weeks before and her physician had advised her that she needed chemotherapy if she was to have any chance of survival. The physician had also advised her of the potential side effects associated with the therapy including the loss of hair, nausea, fever, and immune system suppression with the increased potential for infection.

The woman had consented to the therapy and signed the appropriate forms, but later had begun to have second thoughts. The nursing educator and student had given the patient one dose of therapy when she began to cry and to express her reservations in regard to the treatments. She questioned the nurse about alternative treatments to the use of chemotherapy. The patient related that she had agreed to the therapy because her son believed that this was the best treatment, but she also related that she had not questioned the physician about alternatives as he had already told her that chemotherapy was the only treatment indicated. The nurse did not discuss the patient's concerns with the physician, and later that evening returned to the hospital to talk to the patient about alternative therapies. In the discussion, rather non-traditional and controversial therapies were covered including reflexology and the use of laetrile. The woman's son and daughter-in-law were present at the time of these discussions. During the talk, the nurse made it very clear that the treatments under discussion were not sanctioned by the medical community.

The patient's feelings toward alternative therapies were strengthened by the evening's conversation, but she nevertheless decided to go ahead with the chemo-therapy. The treatments, however, did not bring remission to her crisis, and she died two weeks later. The son who had been present during the discussion regarding laetrile related the conversation between his mother and the nurse to the doctor.

The physician brought charges against the educator for unprofessional conduct and interfering with the patient-physician relationship. The Board of Nurse Examiners for the state of Idaho charged her with unethical conduct and removed her license to practice. An Appeals court later overturned the decision on the basis that the nursing standards used by the board to judge her conduct were too vague, and therefore it was an injustice to remove her license. Although she was somewhat vindicated by the court of appeals decision, the three years of struggle had cost the nurse her teaching position and harmed her career.[9]

Who was right in this case, the nurse who acted upon the changing role of nursing to function as a patient advocate, or the physician, who, following his professional code, could not truly advocate laetrile as an alternative therapy? Had the physician done so he would be violating the rule that physicians only practice medicine having a scientific basis. Laetrile has no scientific basis.

What is meant by the term **patient advocate** in a situation such as this? Does it extend to excluding the physician from conversations that potentially affect the patient's medical decisions? The role of the nurse is changing, but even as late as 1985 two other nurse-patient relationship models beyond patient advocate were still being discussed. Under both of these, the bureaucratic model (where the emphasis is

on the maintenance of social order at the expense of the individual patient's welfare) and the physician advocate model (where the goal is to enhance the authority of the physician), the nurses actions could have been considered contrary to good order.[10]

But what if the appropriate model were that of patient advocate, and the nurse knew that the physician would not have been willing to talk to the patient about her concerns, even if she had asked him? Would that have made the situation different? Would the nurse then have had a legitimate right to provide the information under the requirements of informed consent? Does informed consent require that you discuss treatments without scientific basis?

The fact that the nurse did not discuss the situation with the physician and came back during off-duty hours to discuss the matter with the patient indicates that perhaps she knew that the scope of practice line was being breached. Whether her patient advocate role was such that the decision was necessary is a matter that individual practitioners must answer for themselves. There is a truism that runs "You must not die for principle every day," but every once in a while an issue arises that is of such importance that the professional must not back away even at the cost of his or her practice. The question for all of us is when?

Impaired Colleagues

The practice of health care is often very stressful, and it is not surprising that certain providers have found themselves susceptible to alcohol and drugs. It is estimated that 7 percent of the 1.9 million nurses in the United States today are addicted to alcohol or other drugs, and in one state study more than 90 percent of the disciplinary hearings for nurses within the state were related to substance abuse.[11] These are often very bright, hard-working practitioners who are ambitious and hold responsible positions. What is to be done when you find that a colleague is impaired? Impaired colleagues place clients at risk. The nature of substance abuse is such that even fine practitioners begin to experience behavioral difficulties such as absenteeism, illogical decision making, and excessive errors. Guided by the principle of nonmaleficence, the question that must be faced is not whether the practitioner has a duty to intervene, but rather the manner of the intervention.

The normal questions that one asks oneself are:

- Do I have all the facts?

- Am I sure?

- Is this my problem?

- Who am I to judge?

- Should I ignore the situation?

- What might it cost me if I confront the situation?

- Is it worth the trouble?

The problem with these rather legitimate and normal questions is that they often do not lead to the correct answer. It is too easy to say "How terrible! I'm sorry about —————————, but its not my job to tell anyone." The problem with this ap-

proach is that it is very enabling and does not assist the impaired provider. Equally problematic is the muttering to friends about "poor old Joe," as that is not effective in stopping the behavior and is destructive to the individual's reputation and to the reputation all health care specialists.

Suppose you saw a colleague administer only one-half of a dose of narcotic, place the syringe in his pocket, and leave for the bathroom. To make the case clearer, suppose you later found the bloody, empty syringe in the restroom wastebasket. What should you do? Lets say that you confronted the individual and he denied the whole thing. Addicted individuals often seem to have an infinite supply of rationalizations, prevarications, and subterfuges to show that the truth is untrue. It is hard to imagine a more unpleasant task than confronting a colleague in regard to substance abuse, but—pleasant or no—the health care provider must be confronted and be made to seek effective assistance. Where possible, it is best that the individual be encouraged to seek the help independently; where not, help must still be obtained in order to protect the patients and to salvage the practitioner. Regardless of how the process goes, the basic elements are that the practitioner receives effective help, and that those with knowledge of the situation treat the impaired colleague humanely, as we would any patient who needed our assistance.

WHISTLE-BLOWING

Whistle-blowing in cases where we find colleague or institutional misconduct that must be addressed is often very painful and not always appreciated by the institution one serves. In the book *Secrets,* the author states that the elements of dissent, accusation, and breach of loyalty, common to the nature of whistle-blowing, combine to create an almost natural negative reaction toward the whistle-blower.[12] Hospitals are usually hierarchical and bureaucratic institutions that often do not respond well to whistle-blowing, especially if the complaint is lodged against someone in a higher professional position. Correction of the problem may often cost money, embarrass individuals or the institution, and change the status quo. In that no one likes problems, the messenger is often given as much grief as the person who was the actual problem. Harassment, avoidance, demotion, or termination have sometimes been the fate of those who have reported unpleasant but true instances of misconduct.[13] Because of these potential ramifications the professional must be very sure of his or her ground, gather all the facts, and be able to describe the situation in very concrete terms before taking the problem through appropriate internal channels. Figure 12–3 offers guidance on when whistle-blowing is justified.[14]

Regardless of risk, the professional must also recognize that not to report serious misconduct is to become an accessory to the conduct. Whistle-blowing is a process of gatekeeping, a function of role duty and professionalism that cannot be ignored. Peter Raven-Hansen, an attorney, has outlined a series of defensive strategies for those who have decided that an exercise in whistle-blowing is necessary:[15]

- Write a clear, short summary of the situation, describe what it means and why action is necessary. Once the process is started, meticulous documentation of who said what, to whom and when, is necessary.

- The wrongdoing in question is grave and has created, or is likely to create, serious harm.

- The professional who is contemplating blowing the whistle has appropriate information and is competent to make a judgment about the wrongdoing.

- The professional has consulted others to confirm their information and judgment.

- All other internal resources to resolve the problem have been exhausted.

- There is a good likelihood that the whistle-blowing will serve a useful purpose.

- The harm created by the whistle-blowing is less than the harm done by a continuation of the wrongdoing.

FIGURE 12–3 Justification of Whistle-Blowing

- Avoid personalization; focus on the nature of the incident.

- Where possible, have your statements verified by other health care providers. Sticking to the incident will assist you in avoiding libel and slander charges.

- Make every effort to settle the matter internally. In most cases the media is the last, rather than the first, channel to use.

- Do not believe that you can remain anonymous. The nature of the incident and the details of the disclosure will more than likely reveal who blew the whistle.

- Expect a slow process. The nature of bureaucratic institutions creates an inertial barrier to change.

- Expect retaliation. Disclosures of this nature often are embarrassing and costly to those involved. The whistle-blower must expect to face characterizations of being a snitch, and a disloyal problem-causer. The whistle-blower must be prepared to either live with these attitudes or move on to another position.

Whistle-blowing is not a task that should be entered into casually. Even under the best of circumstances, the individual must understand that, though necessary, the position of whistle-blower is high-risk, often lonely, and rarely appreciated. A quotation from attorney Joseph Rose, whose career was initially placed on hold as a result of whistle-blowing, provides some understanding of the nature of the process.

> Gandhi said that noncooperation with evil is as much a duty as cooperation with good; Edmund Burke said that the only thing necessary for the triumph of evil is for good men to do nothing. Both concepts are still viable . . . although expensive.[16]

Often practitioners are faced with moral distress in that they know what is right but seem unable to follow the correct path. This distress is common among allied health practitioners and nurses, as these health care providers are responsible to many masters. The most commonly perceived constraints are physicians, fear of lawsuits, hospital policies, habits of professional socialization that require the following of orders, and fear of loss of security.

There is a natural ambiguity to the practice of health care that seems to create a certain amount of moral distress. Providers, however, can reduce this by asserting more control over their situation. The first and perhaps most essential form of this self-assertion is to interview potential employers as to their attitudes toward important issues prior to signing on as an employee. Quite often we look only to the pay, fringe benefits, or distance from home in making employment decisions. Equally important would be the institutions' policies in the areas of abortion, euthanasia, incompetent patients, religious matters, living wills, organ procurement, codes, and team medicine.

SUMMARY

This chapter has dealt with several functions that can be listed under the headings of "small ethics." While they do not deal with the great life and death issues such as euthanasia, justice, or withholding/withdrawing life support, they are the daily stuff of modern practice. They come to us as a function of our role duty and are the price one pays for being a professional. As practitioners of health professions we have an obligation to our patients, our colleagues, and our professions to perform these necessary—albeit unpleasant—gatekeeping tasks.

CLARIFICATION EXERCISES

A. In this chapter the authors clearly state that, on an ethical basis, going beyond your scope of practice, having sexual relations with patients, and self-referrals are problems. Write a short paragraph for each of these practices using a legitimate moral rationale (excepting "that's how I feel") indicating why these practices do harm to the professions, the practitioners, and the patients we serve.

   1. Going beyond scope of practice:
   2. Sexual relations with patients:
   3. Self-Referral:

B. In the article (found in the chapter) regarding inappropriate resuscitation, the therapist was attempting to bring about legitimate change in practice. What he wanted, was the establishment of guidelines such as:[17]

   1. DNR orders should be documented in the written medical record.
   2. DNR orders should specify the exact nature of the treatment to be withheld.
   3. Patients, when they are able, should participate in DNR decisions. Their involvement and wishes should be documented in the medical record.
   4. Decisions to withhold CPR should be discussed with the health care team.
   5. DNR status should be reviewed on a regular basis.
   6. DNR is not equivalent to medical or psychological abandonment.

With the above guidelines in mind, first underline the sections within the article that appear inflammatory and devoid of collegiality. Second, rewrite the article so that it is less inflammatory and more persuasive. Third, decide upon a plan (Who, What, Where, Why, When) on how you are going to go about bringing your ideas in regard to changing the resuscitation policy so that it comes into line with the above guidelines.

C. The story in regard to the nursing educator from Idaho was essentially true. Indicate whether you think the nurse or the Board of Nursing were correct. In deciding, use the decision-making model proposed by M.C. Silva:[18]

1. Gather the facts.

2. Identify the dilemma in concrete terms.

3. Explore all options and rules or principles governing each option.

4. Make a decision and be prepared to reflect upon the decision.

REFERENCES AND SUGGESTED READING

1. General Medical Council, *Professional Conduct and Discipline: Fitness to Practice* (London: General Medical Council, 1989), 17.

2. James Whitacre, "Ole Nincompoop Says: Help Stamp Out Inappropriate Resuscitation," *Newsletter of the Missouri Society for Respiratory Therapy* (1980): 11–12.

3. Elton Scott and Mark Ahern, "Effects of Joint Ventures on Health Care Costs, Access and Quality," *Nursing Economics* 10, no. 2 (Mar–April 1992): 101–109.

4. Jean Mitchell and Elton Scott, "New Evidence of the Prevalence and Scope of Physician Joint Ventures," *Journal of the American Medical Association* 268, no. 1 (July 1992): 80–84.

5. Mitchell and Scott, "New Evidence of the Prevalence and Scope of Physican Joint Ventures" (1992).

6. Jerome Freeman and Brian Kaatz, "The Physician and the Pharmaceutical Detail Man: An Ethical Analysis," *The Journal of Medical Humanities and Bioethics* 8, no. 1 (Spring/Summer 1987).

7. American Association for Respiratory Care, "AARC Statement in Regard to Ethical Performance of Respiratory Home Care," Judicial Committee, AARC.

8. Gerald Winslow, from "Loyalty to Advocacy: A New Metaphor for Nursing," *Hastings Center Report* (June 1984), 32–39.

9. In re *Tuma,* Supreme Court, State of Idaho case 12587, 1977.

10. W.J.Pinch, "Ethical Dilemmas in Nursing: The Role of the Nurse and Perceptions of Autonomy," *Journal of Nursing Education,* 24, no. 9 (1985): 372–376.

11. Deanna Alexander and Josie Larson, "When Nurses Are Addicted to Drugs," *Nursing 90* (August 1990): 55–58.

12. Sissila Bok, *Secrets* (New York: Vintage Books, 1983).

13. Morton Glazer, "Ten Whistle-Blowers and How They Fared," *Hastings Center Report* 13, no. 6 (October 1983): 33.

14. Amy Haddad, and Charles Dougherty, Whistle-Blowing in the OR: The Ethical Implications," *Today's O.R. Nurse* (March 1991): 30–33.

15. Peter Raven-Hansen, Do's and Dont's for Whistle-Blowers: Planning for Trouble, *Technology Review* (1980): 34–44.

16. Joseph Rose, as quoted in M. Glazer, Ten Whistle-Blowers and How They Fared, *Hastings Center Report* 13, no. 6 (October 1983).

17. Stuart Younger, "Do Not Resuscitate Orders: No Longer a Secret but Still a Problem," *Hastings Center Report* 17 (February 1987): 24–35.

18. M. C. Silva, *Ethical Decision Making in Nursing Administration* (Norwalk, CT: Appleton and Lange, 1990).

CODES OF ETHICS

American Hospital Association, "A Patient's Bill of Rights"

American Association for Respiratory Care, Code of Ethics

The Hippocratic Oath

American Dental Association, Code of Ethics

American Medical Association, Principles of Medical Ethics

American Nurses' Association, Code of Ethics

American Pharmaceutical Association, Code of Ethics

American Occupational Therapy Association, Code of Ethics

American Physical Therapy Association, Code of Ethics

American Society of Radiologic Technologists, Code of Ethics

American Dental Hygienists' Association, Code of Ethics

American Society for Medical Technology, Code of Ethics

AMERICAN HOSPITAL ASSOCIATION "A PATIENT'S BILL OF RIGHTS"

1. The patient has the right to considerate and respectful care.

2. The patient has the right to obtain from his physician complete and current information concerning his diagnosis, treatment, and prognosis in terms the patient can be reasonably expected to understand. When it is not medically advisable to give such information to the patient, the information should be made available to an appropriate person in his behalf. He has the right to know, by name, the physician responsible for coordinating his care.

3. The patient has the right to receive from his physician information necessary to give informed consent prior to the start of any procedure and/or treatment. Except in emergencies, such information for informed consent should include but not necessarily be limited to the specific procedure and/or treat-

ment, the medically significant risks involved, and the probable duration of incapacitation. Where medically significant alternatives for care or treatment exist, or when the patient requests information concerning medical alternatives, the patient has the right to such information. The patient also has the right to know the name of the person responsible for the procedures and/or treatment.

4. The patient has the right to refuse treatment to the extent permitted by law and to be informed of the medical consequences of his actions.

5. The patient has the right to every consideration of his privacy concerning his own medical care program. Case discussion, consultation examination, and treatment are confidential and should be conducted discreetly. Those not directly involved in his care must have the permission of the patient to be present.

6. The patient has the right to expect that all communications and records pertaining to his care should be treated as confidential.

7. The patient has the right to expect that within its capacity a hospital must make reasonable response to the request of a patient for services. The hospital must provide evaluation, service, and or referral as indicated by the urgency of the case. When medically permissible, a patient may be transferred to another facility only after he has received complete information and explanation concerning the need for and alternatives to such a transfer. The institution to which the patient is to be transferred must first have accepted the patient for transfer.

8. The patient has the right to obtain information as to any relationship of his hospital to other health care and educational institutions insofar as his care is concerned. The patient has the right to obtain information as to the existence of any professional relationships among individuals, by name, who are treating him.

9. The patient has the right to be advised if the hospital proposes to engage in or perform human experimentation affecting his care or treatment. The patient has the right to refuse to participate in such research projects.

10. The patient has the right to expect reasonable continuity of care. He has the right to know in advance what appointment times and physicians are available and where. The patient has the right to expect that the hospital will provide a mechanism whereby he is informed by his physician or a delegate of the physician of the patient's continuing health care requirements following discharge.

11. The patient has a right to examine, and receive an explanation of, his bill regardless of source of payment.

12. The patient has a right to know what hospital rules and regulations apply to his conduct as a patient.

AMERICAN ASSOCIATION FOR RESPIRATORY CARE
CODE OF ETHICS

The principles set forth in this document define the basic ethical and moral standards to which each member of the American Association for Respiratory Care should conform.

1. The respiratory care practitioner shall practice medically acceptable methods of treatment and shall not endeavor to extend his practice beyond his competence and the authority invested in him by the physician.

2. The respiratory care practitioner shall continually strive to increase and improve his knowledge and skill and render to each patient the full measure of his ability. All services shall be provided with respect for the dignity of the patient, unrestricted by considerations of social or economic status, personal attributes, or the nature of the health problem.

3. The respiratory care practitioner shall be responsible for the competent and efficient performance of his assigned duties and shall expose incompetence and illegal or unethical conduct of members of the profession.

4. The respiratory care practitioner shall hold in strict confidence all privileged information concerning the patient and refer all inquiries to the physician in charge of the patient's care.

5. The respiratory care practitioner shall not accept gratuities for preferential consideration of the patient. He shall not solicit patients for personal gain and shall guard against conflicts of interest.

6. The respiratory care practitioner shall uphold the dignity and honor of the profession and abide by its ethical principles. He should be familiar with existing state and federal laws governing the practice of respiratory therapy and comply with those laws.

7. The respiratory care practitioner shall cooperate with other health care professionals to promote community and national efforts to meet the health needs of the public.

THE HIPPOCRATIC OATH

I swear by Apollo, the Physician, by Asclepius, by Hygieia, Panacea, and all the gods and goddesses, making them my witnesses, that I will fulfil according to my ability and judgment this oath and covenant:

To hold him who has taught me this art as equal to my parents and to live my life in partnership with him, and if he is in need of money to give him a share of mine, and to regard his offspring as equal to my brothers in male lineage and to teach them this art—if they desire to learn it—without fee and covenant; to give a share of precepts and oral instruction and all the learning to my sons and to the sons of him who has instructed me and to pupils who have signed the covenant and have taken an oath according to the medical law, but to no one else.

I will apply dietetic measures for the benefit of the sick according to my ability and judgment; I will keep them from harm and injustice.

I will neither give a deadly drug to anybody if asked for it, nor will I make a suggestion to this effect. Similarly I will not give to a woman an abortive remedy. In purity and holiness I will guard my life and my art.

I will not use the knife, not even on sufferers from stone, but will withdraw in favor of such men as are engaged in this work.

Whatever houses I may visit, I will come for the benefit of the sick, remaining free of all intentional injustices, of all mischief and in particular of sexual relations with both male and female persons, be they free or slaves.

What I may see or hear in the course of the treatment or even outside of the treatment in regard to the life of men, which on no account one must noise abroad, I will keep to myself holding such things shameful to be spoken about.

If I fulfill this oath and do not violate it, may it be granted to me to enjoy life and art, being honored with fame among all men for all time to come; if I transgress it and swear falsely, may the opposite of all this be my lot.

AMERICAN DENTAL ASSOCIATION CODE OF ETHICS

Patient Selection

While dentists, in serving the public, may exercise reasonable discretion in selecting patients for their practices, dentists shall not refuse to accept patients into their practice or deny dental service to patients because of the patient's race, creed, color, sex, or national origin.

Patient Records

Dentist are obliged to safeguard the confidentiality of patient records. Dentists shall maintain patient records in a manner consistent with the protection of the welfare of the patient. Upon request of a patient or another dental practitioner, dentists shall provide any information that will be beneficial for the future treatment of that patient.

Community Service

Since dentists have an obligation to use their skills, knowledge, and experience for the improvement of the dental health of the public and are encouraged to be leaders in their community, dentists in such service shall conduct themselves in such a manner as to maintain or elevate the esteem of the profession.

Emergency Service

Dentists shall be obliged to make reasonable arrangements for the emergency care of their patients of record. Dentists shall be obliged when consulted in an emergency by patients not of record to make reasonable arrangements for emergency care. If treatment is provided, the dentist, upon completion of such treatment, is obliged to return the patient to his or her regular dentist unless the patient expressly reveals a different preference.

Consultation and Referral

Dentist shall be obliged to seek consultation, if possible, whenever the welfare of patients will be safeguarded or advanced by utilizing those who have special skills, knowledge, and experience. When patients visit or are referred to specialists or consulting dentists for consultation:

1. The specialists or consulting dentists upon completion of their care shall return the patient, unless the patient expressly reveals a different preference, to the referring dentist, or if none, to the dentist of record for future care.
2. The specialists shall be obliged when there is no referring dentist and upon a completion of their treatment to inform patients when there is a need for further dental care.

Use of Auxiliary Personnel

Dentists shall be obliged to protect the health of their patient by only assigning to qualified auxiliaries those duties which can be legally delegated. Dentists shall be further obliged to prescribe and supervise the work of all auxiliary personnel working under their direction and control.

Justifiable Criticism

Dentists shall be obliged to report to the appropriate reviewing agency as determined by the local component or constituent society instances of gross or continual faulty treatment by other dentists.

Patients should be informed of their present oral health status without disparaging comment about prior services.

Dentists issuing a public statement with respect to the profession shall have a reasonable basis to believe that the comments made are true.

Expert Testimony

Dentists may provide expert testimony when that testimony is essential to a just and fair disposition of a judicial or administrative action.

Rebate and Split Fees

Dentists shall not accept or tender "rebates" or "split fees."

Representation of Care

Dentists shall not represent the care being rendered to their patients in a false or misleading manner.

Representation of Fees

Dentists shall not represent the fees being charged for providing care in a false or misleading manner.

Education

The privilege of dentists to be accorded professional status rests primarily in the knowledge, skill, and experience with which they serve their patients and society. All dentists, therefore, have the obligation of keeping their knowledge and skill current.

Government of a Profession

Every profession owes society the responsibility to regulate itself. Such regulation is achieved largely through the influence of the professional societies. All dentists, therefore, have the dual obligation of making themselves a part of a professional society and of observing its rules of ethics.

Research and Development

Dentists have the obligation of making the results and benefits of their investigative efforts available to all when they are useful in safeguarding or promoting the health of the public.

Devices and Therapeutic Methods

Except for formal investigative studies, dentists shall be obliged to prescribe, dispense, or promote only those devices, drugs, and other agents whose complete formulae are available to the dental profession. Dentist shall have the further obligation of not holding out as exclusive any device, agent, method, or technique.

Patents and Copyrights

Patents and copyrights may be secured by dentists provided that such patents and copyrights shall not be used to restrict research or practice.

Professional Announcement

In order to properly serve the public, dentists should represent themselves in a manner that contributes to the esteem of the profession. Dentists should not misrepresent their training and competence in any way that would be false or misleading in any material respect.

Advertising

Although any dentist may advertise, no dentist shall advertise or solicit patients in any form of communication in a manner that is false or misleading in any material respect.

Name of Practice

Since the name under which a dentist conducts his or her practice may be a factor in the selection process of the patient, the use of a trade name or an assumed name that is false or misleading in any material respect is unethical.

Use of the name of a dentist no longer actively associated with the practice may be continued for a period not to exceed one year.

Announcement of Specialization and Limitation of Practice

This section is designed to help the public make an informed selection between the practitioner who has completed an accredited program beyond the dental degree and a practitioner who has not completed such a program.

The special areas of dental practice approved by the American Dental Association and the designation for ethical specialty announcement and limitation of practice are: dental public health, endodontics, oral pathology, oral and maxillofacial surgery, orthodontics, pediatric dentistry, periodontics, and prosthodontics.

Dentists who choose to announce specialization should use "specialist in" or "practice limited to" and shall limit their practice exclusively to the announced special area(s) of dental practice, provided at the time of the announcement such dentists have met in each approved specialty for which they announce the existing educational requirements and standards set forth by the American Dental Association.

Dentists who use their eligibility to announce as specialists to make the public believe that specialty services rendered in the dental office are being rendered by qualified specialists when such is not the case are engaged in unethical conduct. The burden of responsibility is on specialists to avoid any inference that general practitioners who are associated with specialists are qualified to announce themselves as specialists.

General Standards

The following are included within the standards of the American Dental Association for determining the education, experience, and other appropriate requirements for announcing specialization and limitation of practice:

1. The special area(s) of dental practice and an appropriate certifying board must be approved by the American Dental Association.

2. Dentists who announce as specialists must have successfully completed an educational program accredited by the Commission on Dental Accreditation, two or more years in length, as specified by the Council on Dental Education, or be diplomates of an American Dental Association recognized certifying board. The scope of the individual specialist's practice shall be governed by the educational standards for the specialty in which the specialist is announcing.

3. The practice carried on by dentists who announce as specialists shall be limited exclusively to the special area(s) of dental practices announced by the dentist.

Standards for Multiple-Specialty Announcements

Educational criteria for announcement by dentists in additional recognized specialty areas are the successful completion of an educational program accredited by the Commission on Dental Accreditation in each area for which the dentist wishes to announce.

Dentists who completed their advanced education in programs listed by the Council on Dental Education prior to the initiation of the accreditation process in 1967 and who are currently ethically announcing as specialists in a recognized area may announce in additional areas provided they are educationally qualified or are certified diplomates in each area for which they wish to announce. Documentation of successful completion of the educational program(s) must be submitted to the appropriate constituent society. The documentation must assure that the duration of the program(s) is a minimum of two years except for oral and maxillofacial surgery which must have been a minimum of three years in duration.

General Practitioner Announcement of Services

General dentists who wish to announce the services available in their practices are permitted to announce the availability of those services so long as they avoid any communications that express or imply specialization. General dentists shall also state that the services are being provided by general dentists. No dentist shall announce available services in any way that would be false or misleading in any material respect.

Chemical Dependency

It is unethical for a dentist to practice while abusing controlled substances, alcohol, or other chemical agents which impair the ability to practice. All dentists have an ethical obligation to urge impaired colleagues to seek treatment. Dentists with first-hand knowledge that a colleague is practicing dentistry when so impaired have an ethical responsibility to report such evidence to the professional assistance committee of a dental society.

AMERICAN MEDICAL ASSOCIATION PRINCIPLES OF MEDICAL ETHICS

Preamble

The medical profession has long subscribed to a body of ethical statements developed primarily for the benefit of the patient. As a member of this profession, a physician must recognize responsibility not only to patients, but also to society, to other health professionals, and to self. The following principles adopted by the American Medical Association are not laws, but standards of conduct which define the essentials of honorable behavior for the physician.

1. A physician shall be dedicated to providing competent medical service with compassion and respect for human dignity.

2. A physician shall deal honestly with patients and colleagues, and strive to expose those physicians deficient in character or competence, or who engage in fraud or deception.

3. A physician shall respect the law and also recognize a responsibility to seek changes in those requirements which are contrary to the best interests of the patient.

4. A physician shall respect the rights of patients, of colleagues, and of other health professionals, and shall safeguard patient confidences within the constraints of the law.

5. A physician shall continue to study, apply and advance scientific knowledge, make relevant information available to patients, colleagues, and the public, obtain consultation, and use the talents of other health professionals when indicated.

6. A physician shall, in the provision of appropriate care, except in emergencies, be free to choose whom to serve, with whom to associate, and the environment in which to provide medical services.

7. A physician shall recognize a responsibility to participate in activities contributing to an improved community.

AMERICAN NURSE'S ASSOCIATION CODE OF ETHICS

1. The nurse provides services with respect for human dignity and the uniqueness of the client, unrestricted by considerations of social or economic status, personal attributes, or the nature of health problems.

2. The nurse safeguards the client's right to privacy by judiciously protecting information of a confidential nature.

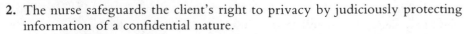

3. The nurse acts to safeguard the client and the public when health care and safety are affected by the incompetent, unethical, or illegal practice of any person.

4. The nurse assumes responsibility and accountability for individual nursing judgments and actions.

5. The nurse maintains competence in nursing.

6. The nurse exercises informed judgment and uses individual competence and qualifications as criteria in seeking consultation, accepting responsibilities, and delegating nursing activities to others.

7. The nurse participates in activities that contribute to the ongoing development of the profession's body of knowledge.

8. The nurse participates in the profession's efforts to implement and improve standards of nursing.

9. The nurse participates in the profession's efforts to establish and maintain conditions of employment conducive to high-quality nursing care.

10. The nurse participates in the profession's effort to protect the public from misinformation and misrepresentation and to maintain the integrity of nursing.

11. The nurse collaborates with members of the health professions and other citizens in promoting community and national efforts to meet the health needs of the public.

AMERICAN PHARMACEUTICAL ASSOCIATION CODE OF ETHICS

These principles of professional conduct for pharmacists are established to guide the pharmacist in his relationship with patients, fellow practitioners, other health professionals, and the public.

A Pharmacist should hold the health and safety of patients to be of first consideration; he should render to each patient the full measure of his ability as an essential health practitioner.

A Pharmacist should never knowingly condone the dispensing, promoting, or distributing of drugs or medical devices, or assist therein, which are not of good quality, which do not meet standards required by law, or which lack therapeutic value for the patient.

A Pharmacist should always strive to perfect and enlarge his professional knowledge. He should utilize and make available this knowledge as may be required in accordance with his best professional judgment.

A Pharmacist has the duty to observe the law, to uphold the dignity and honor of the profession, and to accept its ethical principles. He should not engage in any activity that will bring discredit to the profession and should expose, without fear or favor, illegal or unethical conduct in the profession.

A Pharmacist should seek at all times only fair and reasonable remuneration for his services. He should never agree to, or participate in, transactions with practitioners of other health professions or any other person under which fees are divided or which may cause financial or other exploitation in connection with the rendering of his professional services.

A Pharmacist should respect the confidential and personal nature of his professional records; except where the best interest of the patient requires or the law demands, he should not disclose such information to anyone without proper patient authorization.

A Pharmacist should not agree to practice under terms or conditions which tend to interfere with or impair the proper exercise of his professional judgment and skill, which tend to cause a deterioration of the quality of his service, or which require him to consent to unethical conduct.

A Pharmacist should strive to provide information to patients regarding professional services truthfully, accurately, and fully and should avoid misleading patients regarding the nature, cost, or value of the pharmacist's professional services.

A Pharmacist should associate with organizations having for their objective the betterment of the profession of pharmacy; he should contribute of his time and funds to carry on the work of these organizations.

AMERICAN OCCUPATIONAL THERAPY ASSOCIATION CODE OF ETHICS

Principle 1 (Beneficence/Autonomy)

Occupational therapy personnel shall demonstrate a concern for the welfare and dignity of the recipient of their services.

   A. The individual is responsible for providing services without regard to race, creed, national origin, sex, age, handicap, disease entity, social status, financial status, or religious affiliation.

   B. The individual shall inform those people served of the nature and potential outcomes of treatment and shall respect the right of potential recipients of service to refuse treatment.

   C. The individual shall inform subjects involved in education or research activities of the potential outcome of those activities.

   D. The individual shall include those people served in the treatment planning process.

   E. The individual shall maintain goal-directed and objective relationships with all people served.

F. The individual shall protect the confidential nature of information gained from educational, practice, and investigational activities unless sharing such information could be deemed necessary to protect the well-being of a third party.

G. The individual shall take all reasonable precautions to avoid harm to the recipient of services or detriment to the recipient's property.

H. The individual shall establish fees, based on cost analysis, that are commensurate with services rendered.

Principle 2 (Competence)

Occupational therapy personnel shall actively maintain high standards of professional competence.

A. The individual shall hold the appropriate credential for providing service.

B. The individual shall recognize the need for competence and shall participate in continuing professional development.

C. The individual shall function within the parameters of his or her competence and the standards of the profession.

D. The individual shall refer clients to other service providers or consult with other service providers when additional knowledge and expertise is required.

Principle 3 (Compliance With Laws and Regulations)

Occupational therapy personnel shall comply with laws and Association policies guiding the profession of occupational therapy.

A. The individual shall be acquainted with applicable local, state, federal, and institutional rules and Association policies and shall function accordingly.

B. The individual shall inform employers, employees, and colleagues about those laws and policies that apply to the profession of occupational therapy.

C. The individual shall require those whom they supervise to adhere to the Code of Ethics.

D. The individual shall accurately record and report information.

Principle 4 (Public Information)

Occupational therapy personnel shall provide accurate information concerning occupational therapy services.

A. The individual shall accurately represent his or her competence and training.

B. The individual shall not use or participate in the use of any form of communication that contains a false, fraudulent, deceptive, or unfair statement of claim.

Principle 5 (Professional Relationships)

Occupational therapy personnel shall function with discretion and integrity in relations with colleagues and other professionals, and shall be concerned with the quality of their services.

- **A.** The individual shall report illegal, incompetent, and/or unethical practice to the appropriate authority.
- **B.** The individual shall not disclose privileged information when participating in reviews of peers, programs, or systems.
- **C.** The individual who employs or supervises colleagues shall provide appropriate supervision, as defined in AOTA guidelines or state laws, regulations, and institutional policies.
- **D.** The individual shall recognize the contributions of colleagues when disseminating professional information.

Principle 6 (Professional Conduct)

Occupational therapy personnel shall not engage in any form of conduct that constitutes a conflict of interest or that adversely reflects on the profession.

AMERICAN PHYSICAL THERAPY ASSOCIATION CODE OF ETHICS

Preamble

This Code of Ethics sets forth ethical principles for the physical therapy profession. Members of this profession are responsible for maintaining and promoting ethical practice. This Code of Ethics, adopted by the American Physical Therapy Association, shall be binding on physical therapists who are members of the Association.

Principle 1. Physical therapists respect the rights and dignity of all individuals.

Principle 2. Physical therapists comply with the laws and regulations governing the practice of physical therapy.

Principle 3. Physical therapists accept responsibility for the exercise of sound judgment.

Principle 4. Physical therapists maintain and promote high standards for physical therapy practice, education, and research.

Principle 5. Physical therapists seek remuneration for their services that is deserved and reasonable.

Principle 6. Physical therapists provide accurate information to the consumer about the profession and about those services they provide.

Principle 7. Physical therapists accept responsibility to protect the public and the profession from unethical, incompetent, or illegal acts.

Principle 8. Physical therapists participate in efforts to address the health needs of the public.

AMERICAN SOCIETY OF RADIOLOGIC TECHNOLOGISTS CODE OF ETHICS

1. The Radiologic Technologist conducts himself/herself in a professional manner, responds to patient needs, and supports colleagues and associates in providing quality patient care.

2. The Radiologic Technologist acts to advance the principal objective of the profession to provide services to humanity with full respect for the dignity of mankind.

3. The Radiologic Technologist delivers patient care and service unrestricted by concerns of personal attributes or the nature of the disease or illness, and without discrimination, regardless of sex, race, creed, religion, or socio-economic status.

4. The Radiologic Technologist practices technology founded upon theoretical knowledge and concepts, utilizes equipment and accessories consistent with the purposes for which they have been designed, and employs procedures and techniques appropriately.

5. The Radiologic Technologist assesses situations, exercises care, discretion and judgment, assumes responsibility for professional decisions, and acts in the best interest of the patient.

6. The Radiologic Technologist acts as an agent through observation and communication to obtain pertinent information for the physician to aid in the diagnosis and treatment management of the patient, and recognizes that interpretation and diagnosis are outside the scope of practice for the profession.

7. The Radiologic Technologist utilizes equipment and accessories, employs techniques and procedures, performs services in accordance with an accepted standard of practice, and demonstrates expertise in limiting the radiation exposure to the patient, self, and other members of the health care team.

8. The Radiologic Technologist practices ethical conduct appropriate to the profession, and protects the patient's right to quality radiologic technology care.

9. The Radiologic Technologist respects confidences entrusted in the course of professional practice, protects the patient's right to privacy, and reveals confidential information only as required by law or to protect the welfare of the individual or the community.

10. The Radiologic Technologist continually strives to improve knowledge and skills by participating in educational and professional activities, sharing knowledge with colleagues, and investigating new and innovative aspects of professional practice. One means available to improve knowledge and skills is through professional continuing education.

AMERICAN DENTAL HYGIENISTS' ASSOCIATION CODE OF ETHICS

To provide oral health care utilizing highest professional knowledge, judgment, and ability.

To serve all patients without discrimination.

To hold professional relationships in confidence.

To utilize every opportunity to increase public understanding of oral health practices.

To generate public confidence in members of the dental health professions.

To cooperate with all health professions in meeting the health needs of the public.

To recognize and uphold the laws and regulations governing this profession.

To participate responsibly in this professional association and uphold its purpose.

To maintain professional competence through continuing education.

To exchange professional knowledge with other health professions.

To represent dental hygiene with high standards of personal conduct.

AMERICAN SOCIETY FOR MEDICAL TECHNOLOGY CODE OF ETHICS

Preamble

The code of Ethics of the American Society for Medical Technology (ASMT) sets forth the principles and standards by which clinical laboratory professionals practice their profession.

The professional conduct of clinical laboratory professionals is based on the following duties and principles:

I. Duty to the Patient

Clinical laboratory professionals are accountable for the quality and integrity of the laboratory services they provide. This obligation includes continuing competence in both judgment and performance as individual practitioners, as well as in striving to safeguard the patient from incompetent or illegal practice by others.

Clinical laboratory professionals maintain high standards of practice and promote the acceptance of such standards at every opportunity. They exercise sound judgment in establishing, performing, and evaluating laboratory testing.

Clinical laboratory professionals perform their services with regard for the patient as an individual, respecting his or her right to confidentiality, the uniqueness of his or her needs, and his or her right to timely access to needed services. Clinical laboratory professionals provide accurate information to others about the services they provide.

II. Duty to Colleagues and the Profession

Clinical laboratory professionals accept responsibility to individually contribute to the advancement of the profession through a variety of activities. These activities include contributions to the body of knowledge of the profession; establishing and implementing high standards of practice and education; seeking fair socioeconomic working conditions for themselves and other members of the profession; and holding their colleagues and the profession in high regard and esteem.

Clinical laboratory professionals actively strive to establish insightful working relationships with other health professionals, keeping in mind their primary objective to ensure a high standard of care for the patients they serve.

III. Duty to Society

Clinical laboratory professionals share with other citizens the duties of responsible citizenship. As practitioners of an autonomous profession, they have the responsibility to contribute from their sphere of professional competence to the general well-being of the community, and specifically to the resolution of social issues affecting their practice and collective good.

Clinical laboratory professionals comply with relevant laws and regulations pertaining to the practice of clinical laboratory science and actively seek, within the dictates of their conscience, to change those which do not meet the high standards of care and practice to which the profession is committed.

As a clinical laboratory professional, I acknowledge my professional responsibility to:

Maintain and promote standards of excellence in performing and advancing the art and science of my profession;

Safeguard the dignity and privacy of patients;

Hold my colleagues and my profession in high esteem and regard;

Contribute to the general well-being of the community; and

Actively demonstrate my commitment to these responsibilities throughout my professional life.

Index